DIGNITY AND HEALTH

DIGNITY
and
HEALTH

Nora Jacobson

Vanderbilt University Press

NASHVILLE

© 2012 by Nora Jacobson
Published by Vanderbilt University Press
Nashville, Tennessee 37235
All rights reserved
First printing 2012

This book is printed on acid-free paper.
Manufactured in the United States of America

Library of Congress Cataloging-in-Publication Data on file
LC control number 2012003426
Dewey class number 174.2—dc23

ISBN 978-0-8265-1861-3 (cloth)
ISBN 978-0-8265-1862-0 (paperback)
ISBN 978-0-8265-1863-7 (e-book)

CONTENTS

ACKNOWLEDGMENTS

It has been a privilege to have had time over the last seven years to think and to write about dignity. I greatly appreciate the research funding I received from the Social Sciences and Humanities Research Council of Canada and the sabbatical support provided by the Mary Beck Professional Development Fund at the Centre for Addiction and Mental Health in Toronto. I thank Paula Goering for facilitating a leave I took during the first eight months of 2010 to write this book. I am lucky to have shared this undertaking with a number of talented students: Michael Chan gathered literature right at the beginning. Diego Silva wrote a paper with me close to the end. Andrew Koch made important contributions to the design and conduct of interviews and to the early stages of analysis. Vanessa Oliver, whose engagement was the most sustained, extending over a period of several years, was an indispensable partner throughout the project's data collection, initial analysis, and early dissemination phases. I hope Michael, Diego, Andrew, and Vanessa find some of their own intellectual enthusiasm and their compassion reflected in these pages. I am grateful to the people who assisted with study recruitment—for example, the agency managers who allowed us to post flyers or to use their spaces to conduct interviews. Many researchers and scholars have asked important questions or offered me good opportunities, and in these ways spurred me to do more careful and comprehensive work. I am thinking especially of Vanessa Johnston and Claire Hooker in Australia and Janecke Thesen and Kirsti Malterud in Norway. I thank all the people who attended conference presentations or seminars or my talks to service providers. I'm sure their observations and questions taught me more than I ever conveyed to them.

I have also valued the contributions of family, friends, and colleagues. I would like to single out for special acknowledgment my mother, Dolly Jacobson, who saw from the beginning just how compelling a topic dignity is; Suzanne Ross, who listened so attentively to a synopsis of this book during a long, snowy training run we took in February 2010, and continued to ask about it even after race day; and Dale Butterill, whose question during an early presentation of my work in progress helped open up a whole new area for analysis. My association with Carrie Clark and the other members of the dignity working group at the Centre for Addiction and Mental Health showed me some of the ways in which my conceptual thinking might begin to be made practical. For their work during the publication process, I thank Michael Ames and his staff at Vanderbilt University Press, including managing editor Ed Huddleston, freelance copy editor and indexer Peg Duthie, design and production manager Dariel Mayer, and the two anonymous reviewers whose comments did much to improve my presentation of the material in this book. Finally, I would know very little about dignity without the generosity of the men and women who agreed to speak about it. This book will have been successful if it goes some way toward portraying the resonant complexity of dignity in their lives.

A CONCEPTUAL, PRACTICAL, AND MORAL INQUIRY

Dignity exists in a state of some peril. It can be "taken away." Men and women can be "deprived" of their dignity. The verbs people used when they spoke to us about dignity indicate that these threats come in many different forms. Dignity may be "challenged" or "compromised" or "offended." It can be "upset" or "undermined." It can be "stolen," "crushed," "punctured," "eroded," "stripped," "assaulted," or "snuffed out." In some circumstances, it may be "given away." People may "posture," putting on a dignified face to hide a felt lack of dignity. Yet dignity is also malleable in positive ways. It can be "achieved" (from within) and "cultivated" or "fostered" (from without). Individuals or groups may act and interact in ways that "dignify" themselves and others.

Dignity is a "human characteristic" equated with "real worth as a human being" and the "value" of "being a person." Dignity is "the positive feelings I have for myself," "self-respect, self-esteem, pride," and "confidence and self-assurance." One "has" dignity naturally. Dignity is "inborn," "inherent in everyone," and "something that everybody has inside of them." However, dignity also is something "fluid": it exists in "levels" or "stages," serving as an ever-shifting indicator of "your place in the world."

The word "dignified" refers to the outward manifestations of this human characteristic. Dignity is demonstrated in "poise"—"the way somebody carries their self, their speech." One woman I interviewed described "an image of the person as a whole being . . . standing upright and, and intact." A man offered Audrey Hepburn as the picture of dignity: "The way that she conducted herself—she was graceful, she was humble." Others saw dignity demonstrated in behavior, or "manners and courtesy," and in behavioral control—a kind of stoicism in the face of suffering, and self-reliance under arduous conditions. In evaluating their own dignity and that of other people, the men and women we spoke with emphasized "standards and values." To be dignified is "to follow the same rules" as everyone else, but also to act in accordance with "your morals and what you stand for."

Dignity is not a "commodity" that can be purchased, we were told repeatedly, yet people were acutely aware of the ways in which their material possessions and physical appearance—visual cues like cleanliness, good teeth, upright posture, and neat clothing—figured in the dignity calculus of others who were assessing them. They also often seemed to look to the state of their own possessions and appearance as indicative of "deserving" dignity or of having failed to "earn" it.

In another sense, dignity is an attribute of action—doing something "with dignity." The men and women we interviewed described the ways in which individuals may live (or die) with dignity. They spoke of "being treated with dignity" and "treating others with dignity." At its root, they suggested, such treatment is about acting and interacting in ways that respect "the worth and humanness" of both the self and the other. One man called this "common respect," hinting at not only the presumed ordinariness of dignity but also the ways in which dignity is necessarily something shared, created, and held in common.

Robert Fuller, who writes about rank and its discontents, including the myriad insults and injuries to dignity found in the hierarchical institutions that dominate contemporary society, has described the enthusiastic and heartfelt response of readers to his work, noting "an iceberg of indignation out there of which we're seeing only the tip" (2006, 4). Indeed, concerns about dignity (and indignity) run deep for most of us, and dignity talk is ubiquitous in our cultural conversations.

For example, dignity is prominent in the posted mission statement of Toronto's public transit agency. (Ironically, as it turns out, because in the stories we heard, Toronto's subways and streetcars were prime settings for dignity violation.) It is featured in CBC radio discussions of public policy prescriptions for aging at home. Dignity is highlighted in advertisements for services as diverse as cremation and veterinary care and also in solicitations for charitable donations. The concept dominates the appeals of social movements. The 2011 popular uprising in Egypt was dubbed "the Dignity Revolution." European Union member states use dignity in their discussions of remedying social exclusion; there, the term appears to be a catchall synonym for the rights and privileges of citizenship: voice, recognition, participation, and "dignified living." During the recent economic collapse, the president of the New York Public Library told the BBC about the many men and women who dressed in business attire and came to spend the day in the library's reading room. It was, he said, a "dignified" way of dealing with their unemployment (BBC World Service 2009).

Art copies life. Ben Kingsley's character in the 2003 film *House of Sand and Fog* is an Iranian émigré and retired high-ranking military officer who dresses in an immaculate suit and tie each day before leaving an apartment he cannot afford to travel to his dirty job on a road construction crew. In the German novel *The Reader* (Schlink 1998), the narrator realizes that his former lover, on trial for her actions as a concentration camp guard, is illiterate. Her failure to properly defend herself at the trial, the circumstances of her employment as a guard, even some of her crimes—all can be traced to her attempts to maintain her dignity by concealing her inability to read and write. Dignity is the major theme of Kazuo Ishiguro's *The Remains of the Day* (1989), an exquisite portrait of the English butler Stevens as he looks back over the years of his life in service. Stevens contemplates dignity as an attribute of the great butlers, locating it not in a "good accent or command of language, general knowledge" (34), but in "a butler's ability not to abandon the professional being he inhabits" (42). The great butlers are unflappable and unfailingly loyal to their masters, able to suppress not just opinion but any personal feeling. Stevens's tragedy turns out to be that what he understood as dignity was only the embodiment of his own co-optation by the class system. When, late in the novel, he is confronted by a new generation of servants and their more democratic ideas about the meaning of dignity, he realizes the indignity of his own life: by always trusting in his master, "[I] can't even say I made my own mistakes" (243).

Humorist Lynne Truss's (2005) rumination on modern (bad) manners explores another cultural preoccupation, the relationship between dignity and the ways we treat one another: "The crying shame about modern rudeness is that it's such a terrible missed opportunity for a different kind of manners—manners based, for the first time, not on class and snobbery, but on a kind of voluntary charity that dignifies both the giver and the receiver by being a system of mutual, civil respect" (199).

These missed opportunities and other indignities dominate the dystopias we imagine and those we create. In P. D. James's novel *The Children of Men* (1992), dignity has been overwhelmed by a worldwide epidemic of infertility and a totalitarian state that imprisons immigrants and encourages euthanasia for the old. In the 2004 movie *Crash*, the anxious violence of Los Angeles has destroyed the dignity of the city's residents, who seem adrift in a shared nightmare of angry insult. In the 2005 film *Paradise Now*, it is the Israeli occupation of the Palestinian territories that has stolen the dignity of several generations, including that of the young would-be suicide bombers who are at the center of the story. The characters in each of these narratives are damaged; they are subject to and perpetrators of multiple kinds of dignity violations. Their stories revolve around a common plot: humanity's all-consuming fear and hatred prevent individuals from having dignity, but through the courageous acts of an individual, humanity's dignity may be redeemed.

M. F. K. Fisher, who is best (although perhaps somewhat deceptively) known as a food writer, provided in a 1940 letter home to her family an account of a visit to the Mayo Clinic with Dillwyn Parrish, her second husband. (After the amputation of his leg, Parrish was tormented by phantom limb pain, for which the doctors found no solution. A short time later, he would seek relief through suicide.) Fisher's description of the clinic's waiting rooms focuses on the lack of dignity that may be found in hospitals and other health care settings:

> The first two days in the waiting-rooms I was interested in the people, but now suddenly I have looked at them all I want to—or perhaps more than that. The thing that most impresses me about them is a rather pessimistic feeling of their lack of dignity. Most of them are middle-aged or old, and look as if they should have lived and suffered long enough to acquire that clear outline, that repose— that whatever it is that is supposed to show The Dignity of Man. Of

course many of them do look nice, or kindly, or funny, or something. But that isn't what I mean. They are *not* clear, but smudged in their outlines, like a bad photograph which could show their spirits as well as their bodies. They are incoherent, bewildered, petty—and make me wonder what use there is in spending a life without really learning anything. . . . Many of them are ill-at-ease as they go out the big room and grin and blush and pull at their clothes, and look more like self-conscious children than people going to learn about their lives and deaths. (1997, 48–49)

When I talk to people about the subject of my research, they often seem to place themselves in Fisher's waiting room. They tell me about the experiences they or their loved ones have had in systems of health or social care: the vulnerabilities of physical weakness or difference linked to age or chronic illness; the difficulty of finding good or responsive care; invasions of bodily privacy; a lack of clear communication in inter-actions with doctors and other care providers; a mother's struggle to get proper support services for her disabled child; the attention and money devoted to complicated technocratic solutions at the apparent expense of humane treatment; an enduring dignity differential based on wealth or status. These conversations often are marked by anger or sadness, for speaking of dignity can arouse strong feelings.

More formal but no less passionate discussions about these and other aspects of dignity are taking place in the new public health, which is concerned with how a society's epidemiologies of poor health mirror its patterns of social inequality. The frameworks that have been developed or adapted to understand these health inequities and, ultimately, to find effective ways to end them are firmly grounded in a social justice ideology that, while consistent with the history of public health (Rosen [1958] 1993), often has been missing in the individualistic explanations of human behavior that have dominated the field in recent decades. So, for example, we see the capabilities approach—a framework that directs attention to what a society's structural opportunities and constraints allow people to do and to be (Nussbaum 2000; Sen 1999)—turned to examinations of population health (Hall and Lamont 2009). We see a theory of justice elaborated as the moral foundation of public health policy (Powers and Faden 2006). We see human rights principles used to elucidate public health problems, and the design and implementation of "rights-based" interventions to promote individual and collective health (Gruskin and Tarantola 2000; Mann et al. 1999; Yamin 2009).

Each of these newer models for public health theory and practice conceives of health broadly, as a state of holistic well-being and flourishing that is a function both of social conditions and of abilities (or inabilities) to access systems of high-quality health and social care. Too, the notion of dignity is key to all of them, with dignity seen to be either a justification for ideals like fairness and equality, an expressive manifestation of these ideals, or an experiential mechanism that connects a society's achievement of these ideals (or failure to achieve them) and the status of its collective health. Public health theory thus posits a strong material and symbolic relationship between dignity and health: where dignity is lacking, there is a risk for ill health. Conversely, where dignity thrives, so too does the well-being and flourishing that constitutes good health.

The preponderance of research in the new public health (as in the old public health) is quantitative. It uses large databases to measure risk and protective factors and outcome variables and to model the pathways between the two. However, as Richard Wilkinson (2005) has argued, "psychosocial risk factors for disease reflect how we think, feel, experience, and suffer our lives. Understanding them means understanding the social meanings of people's circumstances" (13). The methods best suited to "understanding the social meanings of people's circumstances" are qualitative ones that move inductively from human experience to conceptual categories. In studying dignity, I chose, therefore, to interpret two sources of information about its social meanings: what scholars have written about dignity in the literature of many disciplines and what ordinary people have to say about it in relation to their own professional and personal lives.

Immersion in the literature allowed me to comprehend dignity in one way, and provided an intellectual thread that is interwoven throughout the chapters to come. Talking to people led to another, more grounded understanding that forms the heart of the book. My first conversations, held between the fall of 2005 and the fall of 2006, were with nine individuals working in the field, broadly defined, of health and human rights. I sought out these key informants because of the prominence accorded to dignity in much human rights talk. These interviews focused on their work and the ways in which they and their colleagues understood dignity. I also prompted them to reflect on how the social movements or changes in policy or practice to which they were committed might address this notion of dignity.

Because most of these individuals had already spoken publicly or published on the topics we would be discussing, I always offered them a choice of whether or not they wished to remain anonymous. All but two gave me permission to use their names. Vanessa Johnston is an Australian physician who holds a PhD in public health. At the time we spoke, her research and advocacy work were focused on asylum seekers and the health impact of their treatment by the Australian government. When I interviewed him, Shawn Lauzon was the executive director of the Ontario Peer Development Initiative, which provides support to and lobbies for consumer- and survivor-run organizations in the province. Cathy Crowe is a street nurse and antihomelessness activist. She is a founder of the Toronto Disaster Relief Committee and of Streethealth, an organization that provides health services to homeless and underhoused individuals in Toronto. Mary O'Hagan is a psychiatric survivor activist in New Zealand. At the time we spoke, she was completing a term as a commissioner for the Mental Health Commission of New Zealand. She had also served as a delegate to the body that drafted the United Nations convention on disability. Rebecca Cook is a human rights lawyer and a professor of law at the University of Toronto. Her work focuses on women's reproductive rights. Morris Wessell is a retired pediatrician in New Haven, Connecticut. He has a long history of involvement in innovative community-based practice and was instrumental in bringing the hospice model to North America. Ashok Bharti is the Indian national coordinator of the National Conference of Dalit Organizations and a founder and convener of the World Dignity Forum, a gathering focused on the rights of oppressed and marginalized groups that is held in conjunction with the World Social Forum. The two key informants who wished to maintain their anonymity were individuals who balanced their jobs in health care systems with their passion for human rights, a balance that could at times become difficult.

The fifty-five interviews that delved into people's personal experiences of dignity took place between the fall of 2006 and the spring of

2007. In conducting these interviews, I was joined by Andrew Koch, then a master's degree student in health promotion at the University of Toronto, and Vanessa Oliver, who was pursuing a PhD in women's studies at York University.

Our initial aim for the interviews was to talk to people from a wide range of backgrounds. However, as Andrew, Vanessa, and I began recruitment, posting flyers at community centers and health care facilities, it quickly became apparent that the people who were drawn to the study tended to be those who were in some way marginalized. For example, although I was then working at a psychiatric hospital, we did not make a specific effort to recruit people with mental health issues. In almost all our early interviews, however, the people we spoke to revealed some kind of history of psychiatric problems—a status that, it was clear, was closely tied to their dignity experiences. We turned our focus to finding people who might have lived with other kinds of social exclusion. We were able to speak with people who were homeless and living in shelters, with active users of illicit drugs, with disabled men and women who relied on social assistance, and with a number of economically privileged individuals recently made vulnerable by virtue of age or serious illness. At several points, we sought out interview participants who might answer specific questions posed by our developing analysis. When many people told us that legal aid lawyers were the only professionals to treat them with dignity consistently, we tried to find legal aid lawyers to interview. Similarly, our many interviews with clients of health and social care service organizations suggested to us that to understand how dignity operates in these settings, it also would be important to speak to the providers of such services.

We asked everyone we interviewed to fill out a demographic questionnaire that sought information about age, sex, race or ethnicity, education, occupation, income level, and "any other important ways you would describe yourself." Interview participants ranged in age from twenty-three to seventy-six, with a mean age of just over forty-two. Twenty-eight participants described themselves as female, twenty-six as male. One participant identified as "gender queer." Thirty-three participants described themselves as White, Caucasian, or Euro-Canadian. Fourteen indicated that they were of Aboriginal or African descent. Eight chose other appellations (e.g., human, Canadian) to answer the question about race or ethnicity. (We found that people often had some difficulty answering this question. For example, several people who spoke passionately about their First Nations heritage during their interviews did not note it on the demographic form.) Twenty-one participants had completed some high school or had graduated from high school, while twenty-seven had attended some college or university or had graduated from college or university, and seven indicated that they had postgraduate degrees. There was a wide range of occupations represented. In addition to the professional service providers, we interviewed a number of individuals who were employed as outreach workers or peer support workers to groups of which they were also members. Other people indicated that they were self-employed, unemployed, retired, working as volunteers, or receiving income support. Among the participants who responded to the question about income, thirty-four described themselves as low income (often indicating that their incomes were approximately $10,000 to 12,000 a year), twelve as middle income, and eight (almost all service providers) as high income. The question about "other important ways you would describe yourself" elicited a number of interesting responses. People used the space to highlight the roles that were important to them (e.g., "mother," "married lesbian with children," "storyteller," "Christian"), their notable personal traits (e.g., "dedicated, conscientious," "fun loving and outgoing," "talkative," "well spoken," "intelligent," "nice person, observant," "orange hair"), and their aspirations (e.g., "try to be a good person," "strives for improvement," "would like to be more than I am"). Others used the space to acknowledge darker parts of themselves, noting the particulars of their diagnoses or criminal records.

The questionnaire turned out to be not just a good way of gathering demographic information, but also—through both the answers people provided and the moments of reflection it allowed—an excellent tool for learning something about dignity. One woman commented that her dignity was negatively affected every time she had to write "unemployed" on a form. A man explained that it enhanced his dignity when he described his level of education as "some Grade 12" rather than "just Grade 11."

Doing research in a way that respects dignity means being able to learn from the people we are studying. I admit to beginning this project somewhat cavalierly, not yet understanding the significance of dignity in people's lives. Just after I had posted the first flyers advertising for people to participate in interviews, however, I received a telephone call from a woman who was intrigued by the study and wanted to know more about it, and about me. We spent nearly an hour on the phone that evening, as she challenged my motivations and probed my methods. Eventually she began to tell me some of her stories, recounting several recent incidents in which her dignity had been threatened or violated. She declined to participate in an interview just then, because there was so much going on in her life, but said that she would call back sometime in the next few weeks.

Her phone call was the first sign I had of how this research on dignity would be received. I had been doing interview-based work on topics in health and health care for more than a dozen years and never before had I found people so eager to participate. Never before had I seen such intense concentration and deeply felt emotion during conversations. An iceberg, indeed: everyone seemed to have been waiting for a chance to talk about dignity. The men and women we interviewed persisted throughout the sometimes difficult logistics of making and keeping appointments—often pursuing us when connections were missed or communications garbled. They arrived early for our meetings, prepared with written notes for things they wanted to be sure to say. They raised questions they thought we should be asking and suggested other people we should meet. They used the interview settings to offer us lessons about dignity. (Once, as I was leaving a restaurant with a woman I had just interviewed, the waitress who had served us was standing by the cash register eating a bowl of soup. The interview participant said, "Can't you sit down?" in a friendly way to the waitress, who answered that she couldn't because she was working. After we exited the restaurant, she told me this had been an example of the small ways in which she tries to acknowledge the dignity of others.) After their interviews had been completed, we received follow-up phone calls and e-mails in which people expanded on or clarified points they had made during our conversations. Time passed without further contact from my first caller and I had concluded that I would not be hearing from her again, but she rang me months later, still thinking about the study, now ready and able to be interviewed.

Our final interview question, in which we asked people to tell us how they had experienced the conversation, suggested that these encounters were positive ones for the people who participated. Some liked our willingness to schedule interviews at their convenience and to meet them in the community (practices that were somewhat unusual at the hospital where I worked). Others appreciated that the demographic form was open-ended, rather than being composed of set response categories. We found that speaking about even the most emotionally grueling incidents could be dignity enhancing when the listening was authentic. Several women who cried throughout their interviews told me at the end how wonderful they felt at having had a chance to talk. One man complimented me on my own dignity. When I asked him what led him to make the comment, he told me he could tell I had dignity because I was really interested and had empathy.

Contrary to my initial expectations—I thought I was doing a study of dignity violation—this kind of hopeful emphasis on the ways in which dignity can be nurtured emerged in many of our conversations. While people had no shortage of stories about insults and injuries to their dignity, with a little prompting they also had a lot to say about how dignity may endure or even flourish. Given the difficult lives of many of our interlocutors, the persistence of their optimism about dignity surprised me, and in so doing suggested new interview questions and fruitful avenues for analysis. The richness of people's thinking about personal and political strategies for promoting dignity enlightened me and inspired the parts of this book that explore dignity promotion.

Respectful research is demonstrated in the form and content of its presentation. The first public presentation of the results of this study was at a community forum to which we invited both interview participants and people who had facilitated the research. (When I was called away by my father's final illness, Vanessa stepped in to conduct the forum.) In their feedback to us, people who attended emphasized the subtlety of dignity, urging us to portray it in shades of gray, not stark black and white. They also impressed on us the need to speak plainly about dignity—to eschew academic jargon. Since then, I have presented the study and its findings to managers and frontline service providers at a number of health and social care organizations. There have also been more traditional conference papers, posters, and articles published. The findings have occasioned much thoughtful and sometimes emotional comment from all audiences, as well as some extended correspondence with practitioners and with other scholars—responses I attribute to a growing acknowledgment of the importance of dignity.

In talking and writing about this study, I have tried to do justice to dignity without objectifying, exploiting, or condescending to the people whose lives are the basis for much of what I have learned. I make a point of devoting time to discussions of dignity promotion. I strive to avoid too many absolutes. I try to use plain language. Wherever possible, I rely on direct quotation of the interview participants' own smart, sharp, and often darkly funny testimony (edited for sense and for style—cutting distracting digressions and removing the ums and uhs we use when we speak). One way in which I now know I have not been respectful, and a decision I regret, is my failure to have given all the men and women we interviewed—not just the prominent individuals who were my key informants—an opportunity to be named. Anonymity is the default in health sciences research, but I wish I had offered all our interview participants the dignity of standing by their words.

While "dignity" clearly holds great power—one woman told me, "That word is as strong as love or hate"—I learned from the interviews that the idea is neither clear nor simple. Turning to the literature only complicates things, because there is much confusion in the extant scholarship on dignity. Dignity is variously described as intrinsic and extrinsic, as objective and subjective, as public and private, as unconditional and contingent, as static and dynamic, as hierarchical and democratic, as based on commonality and based on uniqueness, and as individual and collective (Feldman 1999; Nordenfelt 2004; Pullman 1996, 1999; Sacks 2002; Schachter 1983; Spiegelberg 1970). In light of these contradictions, critics argue that the meaning of dignity is so vague and imprecise that the concept is effectively useless, good for little more than clichéd rhetoric and emotional resort (Becker 2001; Birnbacher 1996; Hailer and Ritschl 1996; Harris 1997; Moody 1998). Something about dignity continues to compel attention, however. Thousands of books and articles about the concept have been published in the last few decades. On closer examination of this proliferation, dignity is revealed as an idea with two distinct but intertwined constellations of meaning, *human dignity* and *social dignity*, each of which can be marshaled for different uses.

Human dignity—also called "basic dignity" (Pullman 1996) or "inherent dignity" (Gewirth 1992)—is the value that human beings have simply by virtue of being human. This meaning is understood to be fundamental, axiomatic, and thus the dignity it describes is intrinsic, objective, unconditional, and static. It applies to all of humanity collectively. The question that preoccupies those who are concerned with human dignity is what grounds or justifies this special value? What is it about just being human that confers dignity?

Historically, the earliest justification is a metaphysical or religious one. Human beings have dignity because they are made in the image of God and stand at the top of the ladder of creation, second only to the angels, and because they have been granted dominion over the natural world (Gaylin 1984; Kraynak 2003). God created human nature as a "small world," or a "microcosm" of the universe: human beings contain and encompass all the rest of the creation and its qualities, and thus serve as something of a bridge between God and the other beings in creation (Dales 1977). Dignity inheres in the human soul and in the human struggle to balance sanctity (the upward pull toward the divine) and depravity (the downward pull toward the lower animal life-forms) (Kraynak 2003; Witte 2003).

Giovanni Pico della Mirandola ([1486] 1948) located man's worth in his God-granted "indeterminate nature" (224), which required him to rely on free will and self-determination. Willard Gaylin (1984) argued that "the dignity of our species starts with the Fall, when [Adam and Eve] chose freedom and autonomy, with all of its pains, suffering, and risk—over security" (19). In the writings of Plato and Aristotle, man's dignity—"his distinctive excellence and virtue"—was understood to be his "rationality" (J. P. Johnson 1971, 216). With the Enlightenment, these capacity-based grounds of dignity became secularized, reaching their height with Immanuel Kant, who located human dignity in the exaltation attendant on man's ability to be an autonomous and rational moral agent (Dillon 1995; Hill 1992) as demonstrated in his voluntary "subjection to self-made law" (Shell 2003, 54). This justification allows dignity to belong not just to humanity as a whole, but also to individual members of the species.

Gabriel Marcel (1963) found "the principle of his essential dignity" in "man's finitude" (136). Matti Häyry (2004) later called this the "dignity of sentient beings," noting that "the basis of our dignity . . . is our ability to suffer" (10). In this conception, then, human dignity is grounded not in what raises human beings up, but in what brings them low—inevitable travail and mortality. Humanity's special virtue resides in our individual and collective response to these inevitabilities, a drive "to balance the will to resist (to overcome) with the will to submit (to accept)" (Beyleveld and Brownsword 2001, 50).

A final justification of human dignity posits that human beings have dignity not because of their special relationship with God or their capacity for autonomous moral agency or even their vulnerability to suffering, but because they exist in a web of relationships that grant them value (Malpas 2007; Street and Kissane 2001). We find human dignity "not only in man's essential nature, its ingredients, its structure and its place in the cosmos, but also [in] his values, rights and responsibilities" (Spiegelberg 1970, 61). Dignity "manifests itself in the gesture by which we relate to others to consider them human" (Valadier 2003, 55). Our human dignity is grounded in the simple fact that "we are all some mother's child" (Kittay 2003, 113).

The idea that dignity is "inseparably connected with the relationships between people" (Ritschl 2008, 98) is key to the second constellation of meaning: social dignity. Here, dignity is a quality, a characteristic of individuals and of collectives generated in the interactions between and among individuals, groups, organizations, and societies. Because it is relational, this type of dignity is extrinsic, subjective, contingent, and dynamic. While human dignity is an inchoate principle of value, social dignity is aesthetic (Pullman 2002) and embodied (Street and Kissane 2001), existing in the many and varied forms of expression and recognition of that value (Spiegelberg 1970).

In one kind of social dignity, dignity is a trait tied to an individual's status in the social structure. (This is one of the longest-recognized and most enduring forms of dignity, dating back to the ancient Greeks [J. P.

Johnson 1971].) Lennart Nordenfelt (2004) described this as "dignity of merit," which refers both to place in a formal hierarchy—the "dignity of aristocracy" (Spiegelberg 1970) associated with societies that recognize nobility, and the "dignity of office" (Kolnai 1995) associated with political or bureaucratic systems—and to position in informal hierarchies, such as those constituted by attributes that are widely admired, such as beauty or talent or physical courage, or by the traditional virtues of courage, honesty, or honor (Schroeder 2008). In the first case, because formal hierarchies are by their nature inflexible, dignity is also fixed. In the informal hierarchy, however, dignity can be earned through individual achievement and is thus reliant on continuing effort and subject to constant assessment. In its darkest rendering, this dignity of rank can become "a humiliating form of dignity . . . that is built on a practice requiring the belittling of fellow human beings" (Meyer 2002, 200), a "parasitic" dignity that is dependent on the subjugation—the indignity—of others (Draft Concept Note on Dignity 2005, 201).

The dignity variously called "personal dignity" (Pullman 1996; Szawarski 1986), "dignity of identity" (Nordenfelt 2004), and "dignity-of-self" (Jacobson 2007) denotes what Michael S. Pritchard (1972) called an individual's "sense of dignity," a "concern to achieve and maintain various forms of integrity, as well as attitudes of self-respect, self-esteem, pride, shame, resentment, and indignation" (300). Each of us has an "ideal self" (Szawarski 1986) constituted by a set of personal virtues. One's dignity-of-self depends first on one's awareness of a unique self and then on the perception of a good match between that self and the ideal self. Such dignity is threatened when "the capacity to live by one's standards and principles" (Killmister 2010, 160) is lost, when sense of self is overwhelmed or when "somebody or something forces me to act against my ideal self" (Szawarski 1986, 202). "False" dignity is the product of a particular kind of pretense: a deliberate attempt to cover up a disjunction between the actual and ideal selves (Kolnai 1995).

What we call "dignified" is "the expression of [dignity] in inward and outward behavior" (Spiegelberg 1970, 54). This is a presentational form of dignity (Meyer 1989), sometimes called "comportment" dignity (Schroeder 2008), "an imperative which is articulated in performative language" (Ritschl 2002, 94). The dignity linked to rank is performed through decorous, or appropriate, conduct, especially as it is revealed in encounters between those who hold different positions in a social hierarchy. (It also may manifest as the kind of behavioral adherence to absurd conventions Marcel [1963] denigrated as "a decorative conception of dignity" or a "display of pomp" [128].) Dignity-of-self is expressed through behavior that indicates self-esteem and self-confidence, a manner that balances authority and deference. To be "undignified" is to present oneself in ways that run counter to propriety or that otherwise seem to demonstrate a lack of self-respect. Alan Gewirth (1992) called these the "empirical" forms of dignity because they are manifested through tangible qualities of bearing and behavior and physical cues like appearance and displays of property.

Dignity-in-relation (Jacobson 2007) refers to the ways in which social dignity exists in the dialogues between self and other, between individual and society. In the dignity associated with rank, status or position is dependent on the existence of a socially validated hierarchy. A queen's dignity relies on her subjects' acceptance of the monarchy as an institution and on her meeting their expectations for how a monarch should behave. In dignity-of-self, the notion of having a unique self, the experience of sense of self, the value accorded the virtues that make up the ideal self, and the ways in which these virtues are manifested are all the result of a complex interplay between individual and collective perception. Dignity is a component of what social psychologists call the "looking glass self" (Cooley [1902] 1983); the dignity people see in themselves mirrors the dignity they see in the eyes of those who are looking back at them, which is in turn a reflection of the dignity they are displaying.

The transitive property of dignity—the fact that people can dignify themselves and others—is highlighted in examinations of what Nordenfelt (2003) called the "adverbial" uses of dignity, his term for conduct, like caregiving, accomplished "with dignity." Many authors—particularly those engaged in empirical and applied investigations of dignity—have focused on explaining just how dignity is generated and maintained in relationships (e.g., Chochinov 2004; George 1998; Jacelon 2003; Miller and Keys 2001; Seltser and Miller 1993). My dignity is nurtured by the respect you show me; I dignify myself by showing you my self-respect. I dignify you by recognizing your self-respect; by dignifying you, I also dignify myself. Barry Jay Seltser and Donald E. Miller (1993) sought to explicate this dynamic: "I truly 'have' dignity only if two conditions are met: I must view and carry myself with dignity, and other people must respond to me as possessing dignity" (96). Robert E. Goodin (1981) captured it in one short statement: "The thing to be respected is created by the act of respecting it" (97).

Dignity is reciprocal and mutual, a "meshed dependence of self and others which might also be viewed as a process of collective dignity" (Paust 1984, 167). The dignity of each one of us is dependent on the dignity of all of us, and vice versa. But by virtue of being generated and nurtured in common, it is left vulnerable to threat. "One's own dignity cannot be separated from the dignity that belongs to others. . . . The denial of the dignity of others also involves a certain diminution of one's own dignity" (Malpas 2007, 23). "The dignity of our people must be impaired if the dignity of one is diminished" (Paust 1984, 152). Advocates and activists whose work confronts extreme poverty and other forms of severe social inequality have said, "We all are undignified now" (Sharma and Bharti 2005, 11).

To summarize, then, the literature tells us that dignity has two distinct meanings: human dignity and social dignity. Human dignity is the abstract, universal value that belongs to human beings simply by virtue of being human. As a principle, it admits of no quantity and cannot be created or destroyed. Social dignity is generated in action and interaction. It may be divided into two types: dignity-of-self and dignity-in-relation. Dignity-of-self is a quality of self-respect or self-worth that is identified with characteristics like confidence and integrity and a demeanor described as dignified. Dignity-in-relation refers to the ways in which respect and worth are conveyed through expression and recognition. It also encompasses the sense of dignity as tied to rank or status in a formal or informal hierarchy. Because it is socially produced, social dignity is scalable and contingent: it can be measured and compared, violated and promoted. The two meanings of dignity are complementary in use. The principle of human dignity provides firm ground for the claims of value embedded in social dignity, while the structures and processes of social dignity, so easily identified and described by ordinary people, make concrete the abstraction of human dignity.

This is one story about dignity, and it is a good one. (I have told it often [Jacobson 2007, 2009a, 2009b; Jacobson, Oliver, and Koch 2009; Jacobson and Silva 2010].) However, it elides much of the complexity of the idea, too neatly smoothing over what makes dignity both so compelling and so vexing.

In each of the diverse grounds of human dignity is a tension: the opposite and opposing forces of sanctity and depravity, exaltation and subjection, resistance and acceptance. Similarly, social dignity is characterized by the push and pull between fixity and flexibility, between ideal and actual, between relation to self and relation to others. Both human dignity and social dignity may be made stronger and richer by their ability to accommodate these polarities.

Yet contradiction also weakens dignity. Human dignity presents claims of universality, but the evidence of our eyes tells us that this is not the case: all human beings are not treated as though they had equal worth. Because it depends on a calculation of value, this type of dignity is inherently comparative. Even theoretically, as in its scholarly justifications, our understanding of who or what has dignity is conditional. Neither is social dignity so straightforward. Expectations for what dignity looks like and judgments about whether it is present or absent are situated. That is, they are highly dependent on circumstance as constituted by factors like historical period, culture, class, race, and gender. Understandings of what it means to be dignified and what it means to dignify are always shifting. As they change, they reshape our presentations, our embodied expressions and recognitions. For the very reason that it is social, dignity is always open to interpretation, and thus these expressions and recognitions may be interpreted differently when viewed from different perspectives.

Despite all the neat exegesis, because human and social dignity share a language it can be difficult even to distinguish the two. In particular situations, we are often flummoxed by whether we are invoking a dignity that is inherent, a dignity that is bestowed, or a dignity that must be earned. (Some of the conflicts I will explore later in the book derive in part from this confusion over meaning.) We seem ambivalent about the uses of dignity: at times, we would prefer it to be a commonality that we share collectively—something that brings us together; in other situations, however, we rely on it to be a kind of unique individuality—a justification for invidious assessment and response.

Through its multiple configurations—despite or because of these tensions and contradictions—dignity serves several functions. It is ascriptive, an attribute credited either to select human beings or to humanity as a whole. It is descriptive, adhering to many different kinds of empirical presentation. To the extent that it can serve as the basis for an aspirational social movement geared toward promoting "inflorescent" dignity (Sulmasy 2007, 2008), or human flourishing supported by "conditions of decent existence" (Margalit 1996, 20), it also may be prescriptive.

L ike the people whose voices opened this chapter, I tend to accept that there is something about being human that confers dignity on all of us, individually and collectively—even if I cannot fully articulate what that something is. However, the remainder of this book reflects my opinion that an understanding of dignity is better pursued through the exploration of social phenomena. Although I do return to human dignity in places, my main concern is social dignity: dignity as a matter of expression and recognition, of action and interaction "embedded within complex forms" of social life (Simpson 2004, 187), particularly in the complex forms of our individual and collective health and our institutions of health and social care. I am interested in the ways in which an understanding of dignity may be used to answer two questions: How can dignity be respected in the values and principles underlying health and social policy? How can it be enacted in the design and delivery of health and social services? Because ideas about dignity trace ideas about the proper ordering of society, I do stray from the domains of health and health care as they are traditionally bounded. In particular, I often focus on how dignity matters for people who are excluded from the mainstream because of their health or social status. In this way, the book is ultimately about recognizing dignity as a moral matter, a sentinel that allows us to know right from wrong, and a guide for helping us to act on that knowledge.

CHAPTER 1

DIGNITY VIOLATION
A Universe of Human Suffering

> An exploration of the meanings of dignity and the
> forms of its violation . . . may help uncover a new
> universe of human suffering.
> —Jonathan Mann (1997)

He was a strongly built man whose face and hands showed the scars of rough living. He walked awkwardly, with a limp that seemed to throw him off balance. In telling me about his life he described himself as "a traveler," the son who "seems to stray," and the "black sheep, per se." As a younger man, he "felt that society had just ripped a hole in my heart and I just, I gave up for a while." Time had passed "in an alcoholic haze." He had crisscrossed the country from the Maritimes to the Mountain West, sometimes working, sometimes spending time in jail. He had quit drinking eight or nine years before and now found dignity in being neat and clean and punctual, and in equal regard, "being treated like one of the others." We met in a narrow coffee shop in a shabby part of downtown Toronto, near the men's shelter where he was staying. The shelter was a place where, he told me, "a part of my dignity is being torn away," because he had been accused of selling the painkillers prescribed for him:

> One of the times when you don't feel like you're having dignity is like for example right now, like I'm being targeted because with my medication at [the shelter], they've taken me from getting it once

a day to three times a day, because they said I was selling it. Now
if I was seen selling it, how come it wasn't acted upon at that point
in time? The next morning I wake up and all of a sudden there's
these accusations and then they target me and say, "OK. You're only
allowed to have your medication once every three times a day." . . .
I've got to keep going up the stairs and go to staffing and ask for it
and, you know, I just find that's not right.

I asked him how "being targeted" affected his dignity:

For me, that makes me look like something that I'm not and that
bothers me. It, it's the key: if it goes around to all the staff, then
all the staff are going to look at me in only one way. . . . Even when
they're, they're interacting with me, they're still going to be saying
in the back of their minds, *Can I believe [him] or can I not? He's a
drug dealer.* . . . Now it goes from staff, and staff interact with a lot of
clients and, you know, people just talk naturally and, and then you
start getting all the guys around you saying, "That's a drug dealer,
man." I mean, like, "Stay away from him," right? I just don't think it's
right, and it, it bothers me every day.

It emerged that the new arrangements for getting his medication were
resulting in further injuries to his dignity:

And these guys, they're making it, they're making it worse. Like
having me go up the stairs [which was physically very difficult
because of his disability] or they say, "Well, you can get a staff
[member] and you can go up in the elevator." Well, by the time that
would transact, maybe half an hour to an hour is going to go by.
Now if I had plans to do anything else, they're going to be disrupted
just because I have to wait, wait, wait.

The loss of his reputation among staff members was making it more difficult for him to access the resources he needed:

I have to go an extra two steps than everyone else . . . say, for
getting something. Like bus tickets to get my methadone or go

to the doctor or whatever. It's like I have to go see the worker and then the worker's got to fool around for a little while on the computer and talk to you. Meanwhile, they do this every day, so they know you need it and you have to have it, but instead they've got to hold you there and talk to you about it, and it's like they're just throwing it at you every single day of the week. . . . Well, look at the ticket book, 'cause we have to sign in to get the bus tickets. You can look in there and you'll see my signature's there for the last, whatever, how many days. [But] even then they still give you a hard time and then someone else will come up and bang, "Oh well, I'm going to take care of this guy, give him his tickets." Boom. He's gone. And now like you're still there another fifteen, twenty minutes and, you know, these other people are, you know, listening and they're watching that you're having a hard time. Some people are laughing at you because it wasn't as hard for them, you know? This place, this time is really, really making me not feel well about myself.

He noticed other differences in how people perceived him and how he was treated:

What they're doing is they're dangling this in front of me like a carrot and it's, you know, "OK. If you misbehave we're going to pull this away." And, and the first minute they see any kind of different actions out of me they're going to say, "That's because he sold his meds and now he doesn't have his meds and he's getting all uptight." Or something like that. Which is not the case. . . . They do this sometimes right out in front of people. They don't care. The staff will just get right uptight with you and they'll be loud and they'll make sure that everybody hears and, and, boom, here's the circle and where are you now? You're the bull's-eye.

Like this man, the people we met spoke all too easily about dignity violation. (Some came to the interviews to bear witness to certain kinds of violations or because they wanted someone to hear about a specific, often particularly painful violation experience.) They had large vocabularies with which to describe the insults and injuries to their dignity—

and those insults and injuries were frequent and varied. As one man said, "Indignity has many faces."

Much of the language people used to talk about their dignity denoted its fragility. As we have seen, in the literature, (social) dignity is described as malleable, relational, comparative, and contingent. It thus can be compromised, offended, affronted, or even lost. It appears to be under an almost constant threat. If the recognition and expression of dignity are presentational (Meyer 1989), so too are the "conduct and ideas" (Schachter 1983, 852) that may violate it. These forms of action and interaction are the *social processes of dignity violation.* These processes are of different orders—more or less likely to be part of our common experience, more or less shocking in their severity. I begin by describing those most of us have experienced, then move on to those that are less common and, arguably, more heinous. Initially, I talk about each process individually; later in the chapter, however, I explore the ways in which they often cluster.

The first process of violation is *rudeness.* The men and women we interviewed bemoaned a general lack of civility in social life, reporting that they experienced a pervasive and gratuitous nastiness in many of their casual dealings with others. One man described entering a room and greeting another individual, a stranger: "I just came in. I said, 'How are you doing?' You know. 'I was good until you showed up.' I wasn't expecting that. I just said hi to the guy." Rudeness was common in public places, such as city sidewalks and streets, public transit, and stores. It was often experienced in encounters with individuals working low-wage customer service jobs. The following incident took place in the coffee and doughnut shop that is a Canadian institution:

> My girlfriend bought a muffin, a blueberry muffin. And so she gets it out of her bag and it's half-risen. . . . This side's high and this side's flat and the bottom is pointed and all doughy. . . . So I go to take it back to this woman, this Indian woman behind the counter, and I said, "I'm returning this for another one." "What's wrong?" "Well, it's not cooked, it's not to her satisfaction," I said. "She doesn't want it. I just want to return it for another muffin." And I was very nice. She said, "What kind?" She says, "That is blueberry." And I said, "Yes, it's blueberry, but it's not cooked and

she doesn't want it, so could I please have it replaced with another muffin?" Now I'm getting angry. So she says, "No, you can't have blueberry." . . . I turn to my friend and I said, "She says you can't have blueberry. What other kind do you want?" . . . She said, "I want blueberry." So I said, "She wants blueberry." And she starts ripping me. "It's got [blueberries]! It's got! It's got!" . . . I was totally baffled. I was standing like this. And people were, her manager came out, her manager heard her screaming at me. . . . I ended up getting a blueberry muffin, but it was after a lot of, you know.

People sustained injuries to their dignity caused by the paucity of care, consideration, or heed shown by others. This kind of *indifference* is the next process of violation. A man who rode a bicycle regularly in the city noted, "The traffic out there is crazy. Some of the motorists don't respect you at all. They'll just come right out in front of you or they'll open their car door when you're zipping by and you can get hurt really badly." (The resentment engendered by drivers' indifference toward cyclists may have been a factor in a 2009 Toronto incident in which a bike messenger was killed in an altercation with a motorist; the case attracted special attention because the driver was the former attorney general of Ontario.)

The functionaries who staff the offices of government bureaucracies are well known for their indifference. In settings where health or social services are provided, endless waiting, without explanation or apology, is its hallmark. People who are poor and reliant on a variety of social and health services describe how indifference sends them from place to place in search of someone who is willing to assume the responsibility of doing something: "They can't be bothered helping you or sending you to the right places or giving you the right, the appropriate resources to help improve your life or whatever, you know. They just can't be bothered." The men and women we interviewed called this the "runaround."

A man who works with homeless people in a midsize city near Toronto described a particularly poignant demonstration of indifference:

This was probably the most well-known homeless woman in the city. . . . She was very ill mentally then; she'd been through the hospital system many times and didn't want any more to do with it. . . . She

had breast cancer and she made a decision herself that she didn't
want any treatment, so she died. She died in a, in a coffee shop, just
sitting there having coffee. . . . The staff [member] at the coffee shop
called 911 when [the woman] fell over, but unfortunately she said,
"There's a homeless woman who's passed out here." So she had to
make that 911 call three times over the course of two hours before
an ambulance came, by which time [the woman] was dead. Now
in the grand scheme of things it probably wouldn't have made any
difference—her body was worn out and she was going to die anyway
and she didn't want to die in hospital, so in one sense it didn't really
matter. But the fact that the young staff [member] that called
said "homeless" made all the difference in the world, because the
ambulance would have been there in minutes otherwise.

Condescension occurs when an individual feels she is not being taken
seriously. Her status as an adult is ignored and every facet of her life
is seen to be fair game for cheap advice or control imposed by others.
As one person said, condescension comes from an attitude of "I know
what's good for you better than you do." People described being "talked
down to" or "treated like a child." Conversations in health care settings
seem to be particularly fraught with condescension. Nurses "talk singsong," "like [the patient] is three years old." One man said, "I've had experiences with doctors just saying, 'There's something wrong with this.
I want you to take this drug.' [I've asked,] 'Well, what's it going to do?'
'It doesn't matter what it does. It's going to help you.'" A woman who
was living in a complicated relationship with an abusive partner grew so
depressed and anxious that she had to be hospitalized. As she was being
discharged:

The two women that I talked with were like, "Oh well, yeah, just
throw him out, yeah." . . . And I said [to myself], this is the words of
wisdom that I get from you on my way out the door—oh yeah, just
get rid of him and that will be that. And I was, I was really insulted.
I felt like, you know, just shut your mouth . . . if that's your answer
for me, that's your band-aid for my leaving. . . . I hadn't seen them
before, they hadn't taken any time to talk to me, so they had no idea
really. . . . I mean, yes, that's, that was the best solution but it's not

the most likely one that's going to happen, that's not the most likely thing I'm going to do. . . . The coupon they gave me to leave with was worthless. . . . What they said to me was worthless, it was insulting.

The next process is *dismissal*. People explained that their dignity was violated when their knowledge, skills, perceptions, concerns, needs, or feelings were discounted. A man who described himself as possessing the skills to "build a house with my own hands" told Andrew that his dignity "takes a bruising" when "I'm giving someone information and then, and then it's pooh-poohed. . . . That's like the effect of the opposite of being treated with dignity, you know. . . . You almost feel degraded." A young man remembered an incident in his high school classroom:

We were doing poetry and so [the teacher] read this poem to the class and then asked people what they thought it was about. So I put up my hand and I gave an answer, and she was like, "No, that's wrong." . . . I think it was about like a, it was about something flying, like a bird flying. So I said, "Oh, I think that it's supposed to be about freedom." She said no. [Another student] said it's about flying. She said, "Yeah, that's right." So I said, . . . "Well, isn't the idea of poetry being subjective and that, you know, there's no right answer. It's each reader is supposed to take what they take from it." And she's like, "Well, no, I was looking for the right, real answer."

In health care settings, serious medical conditions go untreated because doctors and nurses dismiss their patients' ability to recognize and report accurately when something is wrong. Having just received a disturbing diagnosis, a woman feels dismissed when the doctor looks at his watch before she can ask any questions. Health and social care providers, on the other hand, report that they feel dismissed when clients ignore their advice or decline to follow through with arrangements they have made.

When people are made to feel smaller or lessened by others or when they report having to "lower" themselves because of circumstance, *diminishment* has taken place. Men and women who were out of work talked about being ground down not just by the fact of being unemployed but also by the process of looking for a job. One woman said,

"Most people who don't have a job, they're the ones that don't have a lot of confidence in themselves after a period of time. They don't get one right away, you know what I mean, and they lose their confidence, you know?" In the offices where people apply for social assistance, "there's a whole culture, a sort of class attitude about dealing with poor people. . . . That's where a lot of the indignity is . . . just that person on the front line who has the . . . check and makes [the applicant] grovel to get it." A man who had spent several months in a psychiatric unit spoke of being diminished by having to lie about feeling better in order to be discharged:

> And the key word is *lie*, because a great many people don't really believe it. But they realize things to say in order to get out of there. So one of the greatest indignities is that you have to not tell the truth to be able to come out. . . . You're not true to yourself. You realize that the health care system is not truly a place where you can be yourself. You have to play the game to get the perceived outcome that both you and the hospital want. It's powerful stuff.

Dignity is violated by *disregard*; that is, when people are rendered voiceless or invisible. Health care providers are often described as failing to make eye contact with or to address their patients directly, confining themselves to conversations with other providers even though the patient is in the room. A transgender woman spoke of the insult to her dignity occasioned by the Ontario government's decision to "squash" public hearings on the amendments to the Human Rights Code without considering the testimony of members of her community: "They stopped that debate and one of the members said, 'We've heard everything we're going to hear.' And I thought that was incredibly insensitive and that was an infringement on human dignity, and the reason I say it was a violation and, and malicious, intentional" is "because they wanted to achieve a particular goal and they wanted to mandate and they predetermined how those amendments were going to take place."

A social worker who provides services to individuals who are homeless described the disregard experienced by street people: "We do not look at the person who's sitting in the corner with their hand out. So just that in itself—somebody to have five hundred people in one morning walk by you, without acknowledging your existence—it's devastating. It's completely devastating. I mean, you're not there. You've become invisible, completely invisible, so that in and of itself is a major loss for any person." And activist Cathy Crowe implied that the invisibility of the individual homeless person is replicated on a larger scale by the increasing invisibility of the entire problem of homelessness: "It's all normalized now. It's all normalized that, you know, we give people sleeping bags outside or people have to line up to get into this thing or people have to line up to do that or we only have two showers for two hundred people. It's all normalized. But if you actually visited from another planet and looked at it, you'd think, 'How can this be?'"

Dependence, whether physical or economic or both, is experienced as a failure and a loss and thus as a violation of dignity. A man who suffered a severe head trauma as the result of a violent act described the loss of dignity occasioned by his injury:

> I'm very independent. I'm a go-getter . . . and coming from that to I want to go to the washroom I had to ring a bell and wait until they come to get me to take me. I want to go have a shower, I got to ring a bell and wait. I want my, some question. I have to ring a bell and wait. That's taking away my sense of independence. . . . That's taking away from me something I always used to have, and it happened just instant. Another thing that hit me really hard about it, because I was on my way to work. My independence to support myself, to support my son, and then all of a sudden—shoo, it was gone.

Dependence runs contrary to the cultural ideal of "self-sufficiency" and the individual's ability to "control [his] own life." A young woman who had worked as an assistant to people with physical disabilities struggled with ambivalence over the dignity dimension of her role:

> Like, it's not OK to be dependent in our society, so you're, so people with disabilities are trying to be helped to be independent, right? . . . But it becomes really difficult when you have to depend on others to get there. So I think it kind of undermines. . . . It was very hard to pin down, but I felt it when I was working, like, with [people with disabilities] that it was because, by virtue of even just helping, that

was a problem, like that made people feel crappy . . . because it's not OK to be helped to get to where you need to be.

Restriction, or the experience of being constrained in one's ability to make one's own decisions and to act autonomously, often accompanies dependence, but it constitutes a separate kind of violation. Restriction is a defining feature of total institutions, like jails and psychiatric hospitals, that impose multiple limitations on their inmates. As one woman who had been hospitalized multiple times said, "They take away your freedom. . . . They take away your clothes. They take away . . ." A psychiatric survivor and advocate for people with psychiatric disabilities reported that in the Toronto boarding homes that house many people who have been discharged from a local psychiatric hospital, residents experience constraints on almost all aspects of their lives: "You're in a place that you have very little control over your environment, if any. You can't control the food that you eat. You can't really control when you wash. You can't control other people's activities in the house." A social worker who provides services to people with addictions spoke of the ways in which drug use itself limits people's choices, but noted that the responses of institutions and individuals to addicts were often punitive and directed at imposing more restrictions. She said, "So one of the issues around dignity is that [this kind of response] makes lives even smaller."

When human beings are treated like things—inanimate, insensate—*objectification* violates their dignity. In health care settings, people are routinely referred to by disease or by room number. During procedures, their bodies are treated as nothing but physical matter. One man talked about bringing his elderly mother to a medical test: "When they take her for X-rays, they treat her like a commodity, and she's given no respect that she's ninety years old, that she's frail, and they were terribly impatient when they asked her to lie on a X-ray table when she can't lie flat." The same man described feeling like "a potato that" a phlebotomist was "sticking a needle in" during a blood draw, while a woman recalled being treated like "a sack of potatoes" during the birth of her first child.

The process of objectification also occurs in social service settings. A resident of the city's shelter system spoke of being nothing more than "a number" to the shelter staff. A woman recounted her experience with an income support bureaucrat: "She didn't want to make any personal connection to me, you know. I'm just an object. I'm, I could be, I could be an object that she's working in a factory and just stamping out the press, you know. I, yes, I speak and I see and I hear but there is certainly no emotional attachments there, and that's hard. It takes the dignity away."

Intrusion is constituted by unwanted transgressions of bodily or other personal boundaries. What should be private is made public; what should be hidden is revealed; that which is meant to be held close is opened up to exposure. Upon admission to a women's jail, "they strip search you and they have male guards walking around in the jail and they stand there watching you get showered." A jealous boyfriend "was always looking over my shoulder and my computer and going into my Day-Timer. Like, I couldn't even write in my journal. . . . That took away my dignity, my privacy." A legal aid lawyer noted the violations of dignity that take place in courtrooms: "What's sort of dangerous in terms of upholding people's dignity, right, in court" is "just the openness and the fact that everybody hears about everybody else's dirty laundry." Despite having ostensibly stringent rules about maintaining confidentiality, social services offices fail to observe them; as one social worker reported, "Your information most of the time is passed to you through this window: 'Mr. So-and-So, your check is ready.' Your name is out there. . . . That information is passed to you very loudly over the window." One person experienced a program offering a particular kind of therapy almost entirely in terms of intrusion:

> [One of the] conditions of the therapy was that all sessions were taped. If you did not consent to that, out you go. And when things got a bit more troublematic, they stuck you in a room with a double mirror. Well, and the therapist wore an earpiece while she was being coached by one of the supervisors as to what to say to me. Meanwhile I'm also being filmed, viewed through a double mirror and being—and then her being coached by somebody who I can't even see. And I had no choice over that. . . . That's an erosion of dignity, freedom of choice, humanity.

Dignity is violated by *contempt*, an attitude of directed and deliberate disdain, which is enacted in word and deed. The two transgender women we interviewed both reported repeatedly being addressed as "sir," an appellation they experienced as an intentional slur. A woman who was beaten while doing sex work found that when "I went to the hospital and they asked me how it happened, I said, 'Well, I was working at the corner of . . .' and as soon as I got that out of my mouth, it was, oh! The whole, the doctor's whole demeanor changed." In hospitals, people who engage in acts of self-harm "are treated like crap. . . . I had a very good friend who ended up in ICU for about six weeks . . . because she had slashed and done a number of other things and the treatment she experienced was horrible, really punitive. 'You're taking up space,' you know. 'Why don't you really kill yourself?' Like just horrific responses, right?" A hospital security guard shouts at a visitor who has angered him, calling her "you big welfare." On the street, a woman is panhandling: "One guy come by me and I asked him if he had any spare change and he asked me why. And I said because this is what gets me my groceries. And he asked me if I was an addict and I said, 'Yeah, I smoke crack occasionally.' And he took a handful of pennies and like whipped them right at me."

The next process of violation is *trickery*, or manipulation aimed at asserting power by making people question their own perceptions of reality. Many people described this kind of violation as "insulting my intelligence." I asked one man, who had used this phrase repeatedly in talking about encounters with acquaintances, police, and the mental health system, to explain exactly what he meant. He held up a blue pen:

> Everybody in this place is telling me it's a fucking red pen. . . . They officially changed the wording from blue to red just because, you know, blah blah blah bullshit bullshit. And you're going, "I don't care if you call it whatever you want." And everybody in the place is going, "Oh yeah, it's red." I don't believe it. All you people expect me to believe this, go out and start going, "Oh yeah, look at that red car" to the rest of society and look like an idiot . . . and they all just lay it on you, "No, no, yeah, it's red." That's insulting someone's intelligence.

(The same man told me that he could insult my intelligence by scamming me for money—by coming back to the study claiming to be a different person and participating in another interview.)

Trickery takes place in many places, including legal and health care settings. A defendant believes that the man who is testifying at his trial is not the witness who was present at the event, although he is being represented as the same person. A man who was left to wait for hours in an empty emergency department said, "Sometimes I think they do it on purpose to see if you get angry, to see if you're a good candidate for anger management therapy. . . . They put you through a whole little test to see if you'll lose your temper. . . . It wears you down." A woman described how trickery was used as part of a specific psychotherapeutic modality:

> They were just trying to, short term, just trying to break, break you. To get you, me, trying to break me to get me to my problem area. . . . This doctor, I'd go in and I'd say hello and he wouldn't, he purposely wouldn't answer me. . . . I'd say, "Can you say hello?" And he'd say, "Why do you need so much attention?" . . . He did eventually get me to tears, you know. But I thought, was that necessary? . . . I just felt like a victim of power.

When people are seen and treated not as individuals, but only as indistinguishable and interchangeable parts of a unit, their dignity is violated by *grouping*. One woman called this "pigeonholing" and described how her landlord had "tried to take [dignity] away" by "grouping" her in with the mass of women—"you girls"—who live in subsidized housing, saying things like "whatever you girls do—go out and have a cigarette or whatever you girls do." Others talked about getting "all grouped together in the one low-life kind of group of people" when they talked to social assistance workers: "You get the impression off them that they think anybody who's on welfare . . . is lacking in some way. . . . It's just an automatic assumption again on the values. . . . [That] if a person is on welfare, that they, you know, there's something wrong with them." Grouping is closely linked with the next two processes of violation, which require that people first be grouped.

In *labeling*, individuals are tagged with a descriptive term that becomes a kind of master status, determining how they are perceived and how they are treated. As a physician told me, certain "stigmatized diagnoses" are powerful labels in the health care system:

> If somebody is, you know, sort of more conflictual or more
> argumentative, they are probably more likely to get a borderline
> personality disorder diagnosis. . . . I see this in Emerg when
> somebody argues with the Emergency staff or with, you know, the
> psychiatrist and gets very disruptive and angry. . . . The human
> response sometimes is to [make an excuse]. Like, *oh, it's not us!* We're
> not failing in our service to you; you've got more of a personality
> disorder.

"Addict" is another such controlling label, a social worker explained: "One of the things that happens in the area of addictions is labeling. . . . [I'm thinking] of, you know, somebody who struggles with addictions, who goes to the emergency for a totally unrelated issue and is not treated because somehow in their chart it says that they are an addict. So, so in that way, it is very limiting and decreases their access to services or in the way that they're responded to by the system."

Vilification is the final step in this trio of violation processes, one that is embedded in the previous two. The process of grouping is also a process of othering—the separation of the "them" from the "us." The labels applied to people often carry connotations of moral deficiency or social inferiority—of dangerous difference. The social worker quoted earlier went on to explain the vilification of addicts that follows their labeling:

> What happens to them? There's a couple of things, in terms of
> the ER. . . . There's a couple of examples that come up for me.
> So one of them is a woman who is in her fifties who is struggling
> and comes into the ER in a state of withdrawal. She's been on
> a binge for a week or more. . . . She's gray, her hair looks totally,
> looks older. . . . She is looking for medical attention in terms of,
> you know, these symptoms of withdrawal, right? She suggests [a

particular drug]. . . . They prescribe [the drug], but at the same time, she's reported to the Ministry of Transportation. This woman has not driven. She's never had a driver's license. She came to the hospital on her own in a taxi, and the assumption is that she's a danger to society. . . . It makes absolutely no sense. It's very punitive.

Once people are vilified, their activities—no matter how neutral or even admirable—also may be vilified. A man who was receiving social assistance told me how damaging to his dignity it was that his (paid) participation in our interview would be maligned as a kind of cheating if his welfare worker were to learn of it:

I'm here more for the study, but the money helps. But I can't declare it to social services. They're going to take it away. I sit there and I look at them and I go, whoa. Here I am doing a good thing and I'm going to sit there and worry about this $25, like a pittance of a pittance in the big scheme of things, and meanwhile they're all worried about that because the system is set up [so that welfare recipients don't even reach the poverty level]. I mean the feeling that you have to hide this stuff away to kind of protect yourself. . . . I would welcome . . . [the opportunity] to go in front of the justice system and say, "You guys sit there and think that I'm doing something bad here, collecting an extra $25 for contributing to a valuable study? Come on!"

Grouping, labeling, and vilification also may serve to further future violations of dignity. Cathy Crowe noted that when Toronto's chief of police made widely reported disparaging remarks about "panhandlers and squeegeers," it "fueled a backlash against homeless people and we saw [violent] crimes increase against [them]."

While dignity is often offended by disregard, it also can be violated by heightened scrutiny, or the social process of *suspicion*. People used the phrase "treated like a common criminal" to describe this kind of violation. A woman who ran out of prescription painkillers while her regular physician was out of town found that when she went to a clinic looking for enough medication to tide herself over, "it's like they're looking down at you and judging you, thinking you're trying to scam something, you know. I'm trying to scam something, you know, like I've got all this stuff and all these [medical] reports and they still think I'm trying to scam a prescription out of them." On public transit, one woman noted, "most people throw in their change [into the fare box] and the driver just pulls the lever down and it goes. [But] people who appear not to have a lot of money, their change tends to sit there for a bit while it's being [counted]." A man who does outreach work with homeless individuals conducted an informal survey of churches to determine what resources might be available to help his clients:

> [I asked,] what do you do if somebody shows up at the door and asks
> for assistance, which is fairly common in the downtown—people
> wanting food or money or clothing or whatever. . . . There was
> one minister at one of the large churches in the downtown whose
> response was, "We don't help anybody who comes to the door,
> because we don't know who's telling the truth." . . . So, you know, I'm
> thinking, you turn everyone away, because there might be one in a
> hundred who might be stretching the truth a bit. Doesn't sound very
> Christian to me.

Suspicion is the hallmark of the bureaucracy that determines eligibility for income support. During our interview, one man imagined how the then provincial minister of social services—a member of parliament from Windsor, Ontario, named Sandra Pupatello—might be interrogated were she to apply for disability support: "OK, your name is Sandra and you're single? Hmmm. And you recently moved here from Windsor? So you're not really living here in Toronto, are you? Hmmm. I'm going to need proof of residency. Can you come back tomorrow to give me more documents? Mmm-hmm. And you're dressed way too nicely, you know. I'm going to have to talk to my supervisor about that."

The physical environments in which these encounters take place can reinforce attitudes of suspicion. As one woman told me, "Any person walking into a [welfare] office is going to be on edge, is going to feel humiliated, is going to feel frustrated. 'Cause everything about that office tells you that. You have to talk through Plexiglas. You're really at arm's

length. Many of the offices have security [guards]. They don't give anyone dignity or respect, right?"

Discrimination occurs when people's rights are denied based on their
achieved or ascribed status or their apparent membership in a low-
status group. Many times, these violations involve barriers to accessing
needed resources, such as housing or health care. One man reported
such discrimination against people with psychiatric diagnoses:

> Certain family physicians are often unwilling now to take on people
> as patients if they're on psych meds. . . . It's very undignified for the
> person because they'll go for an initial interview with the doctor
> and the doctor will ask all these questions and say, "I'll get back to
> you in two weeks whether or not I can take you on." And then more
> often than not there's never a phone call and when [the prospective
> patients] do finally phone, [the doctors' staff] often say, "No, we're
> not able to take her on as a patient."

A woman talked about the discrimination she faces as someone with a
"drug problem": "Especially in the welfare system or the [disability sup-
port] system or any government offices, they find that you have an addiction, they don't treat you very nicely. They don't treat you very nicely.
They treat you like a lower-class citizen, if a citizen at all." This individual found such discrimination to be particularly galling because she
believed many of the welfare workers charged with determining her eligibility were immigrants: "It drives me nuts, you know. I'm a Canadian
citizen and here you are, you've been in this country for a year and a
half, you have a high-paying job, and you're telling me I can't have any
money because I'm a useless individual. It just doesn't sit very well."
Other people described instances of discrimination based on criminal
record, race or ethnicity, gender, and poverty.

The next process of dignity violation is *exclusion*. Here, people are
made to feel shut out of physical or social spaces that are ostensibly
meant to be open to all. A man recounted how he and a friend had recently been excluded at a local drop-in center:

> [A friend and I] walked into one of the rooms that was a Weight
> Watchers room. . . . He picked up a pamphlet and the first thing

[the meeting leader] said, she's like, "Put that down." And my friend said, "Well, we're just looking. Is that OK?" "No. You guys are going to have to leave or I'm going to call security." Oh yeah. It makes you feel unwelcome. . . . [The meeting leader] could have come up and said, "Hi. How are you? Excuse me." You know what I mean? "These products are for the group today." Or see if you wanted to join the group. Or, you know what I mean, something like that . . . but they didn't. They just, you know, "Get out of here. We're going to call security on you." . . . The doors are wide open to the public . . . [but] then once you get in there, you're treated like you don't belong, you know what I mean? You shouldn't be there, just because you're, I don't know, the way, the way we were dressed. I don't know what it was.

A woman blamed the problems faced by Canada's Aboriginal communities on a broader social exclusion, saying, "If you get outside that social basket, there's no acceptance. . . . They're excluded and what's happened, they're dying. They're all dying, you know, they're committing suicide. . . . You know why? Because their dignity has been taken away."

In *exploitation*, people are viewed only instrumentally, as the means to achieve a desired end. Drug-involved individuals offered many examples of being exploited and of exploiting others. (They saw both acts as dignity violations.) A man noted how addicts "use" one another, describing how he had many friends when he was flush with drugs or money, but those friends disappeared once the spree was over. A number of the people we interviewed held up prostitution as the ultimate form of exploitation, often offering it as an example of a line they hadn't crossed: women would state that they had never sucked "some cock for some rock," and men that they had "not once [got] any one of these girls down here to go do prostitution." A man who wore a prosthetic leg reported that he often panhandled in the park to get money for drugs, but was appalled when "one night I took my prosthetic leg off. I was drying it off, 'cause it sweats. A lady gave me ten bucks and I went, 'Oh my God.' . . . [The people who benefited from the cash he had collected] are going, 'You should go panhandling and take the leg off.' And I'm not doing, I'm not doing that. That would be just a pure shame, you know?"

Another man argued that the exploitation engaged in by drug users was secondary to the exploitation of drug users engendered by public policy toward drugs:

> A person who's, who's a druggie hasn't lost their dignity because they're a druggie, to me. I mean, they've made a choice in life. . . . They lose it when they give up food or clothing or shelter or other things to pay for the drugs, just because it's illegal, you know? And to me, that's where the harm comes in. . . . It's exploiting them. So that's where the loss of dignity to me comes in: the fact that it's illegal is what makes it undignified.

Revulsion occurs when people draw back from someone as though he is disgusting or somehow tainted. A woman told Vanessa that because people had recoiled from touching her hand so often—"they look at me and they see AIDS or something"—she now used a paper cup when she panhandled. Homeless people riding public transit also experience this kind of revulsion:

> People come in. They want a seat and you will see them sit down and then you see that person whom they're sitting next to is not very well dressed, may have a body odor of some sort, and people's expressions will be really, really poor. Very badly behaved. I mean, I'm not, I don't ask people to sit next to somebody whose body odor is offensive, but one does not need to make a face and make a big huge drama about how they're leaving that space because that person has body odor.

A man goes to the hospital with a cyst that has burst:

> [The doctor] said, "Well, let me see what I can do." OK, thank you. He put me on a gurney and he looked at my arm and he took the dressing off. He goes, "Oh, that stinks!" And walked away. I never seen the guy again for like twenty more minutes. I said, "What happened to you?" when he came back. He said, "Oh, the stink was unbearable. I had to leave." I said, "But sir, you're a doctor."

Dignity is violated when people lack the basic necessities of life—clothing, food, shelter, or health care. "Dignity is all wrapped up as a part and parcel of what comes with the territory of either having those needs met or having those needs not met," said one man. Such *deprivation* may be either relative or absolute. The same man continued, "It's impossible to have dignity in an under-resourced and under-recognized environment . . . any kind of social environment where people have things and other people don't have things." For people who are homeless, another man told me, "there's little situations each and every day that confirm the fact that you aren't worth a shit":

> You can't get a family doctor. You can't afford to buy your own food. You have to go to the drop-ins and the shelters and to wherever else where there are community meals. You know you're supposed to be on this special diet but you can't do it, you know. . . . You can't buy the stuff that you're supposed to be eating, so you have to eat what you're given, so that must mean you're really not worth a shit. I don't know. There's countless ways. You, you can't afford transportation, you know, and it's very embarrassing to panhandle.

The social safety net is inadequate to deal with the dignity violation attendant on deprivation. Instead, bureaucratic policies and procedures seem to exacerbate violation, sending a message that "people on welfare have less value than somebody else."

One woman defined *bullying* as "dominating or trying to control someone to make somebody, to make themselves look good or look better or whatever." Bullying encompasses mockery, threats, and both physical menacing and psychological intimidation. The bully "gets in [people's] faces," seeking to "put them down." One man talked about being bullied regularly in high school: "In school I was picked on a lot and beaten up. . . . A bunch of guys that thought they were really tough decided that I was gay. So it was, you know, a good thing to do, you know, to make fun of me and kind of push me around and beat me up a little bit. So, you know, it's hard to keep your dignity intact when that's going on." A man described being bullied by his landlord, a "notorious slumlord":

[He] really seems to have a good time trying to put me down and making me feel bad. . . . One day he came into my house and he went right into my room without asking. He grabbed all my possessions and threw them out on the street. He said, "If you don't pay, you don't stay." I asked him for an eviction notice. He still has yet to file an eviction notice. He just keeps coming down with, with people I've never even met before, threatening me, intimidating me. He tried to scare me out of the house. And so, you know, he can really bring me down. He scares me, you know. He struck me a couple of times. He's pushed me around a few times, and he's thrown my belongings right on the street. And that really makes me feel bad. Makes me feel like I'm doing something wrong.

Assault is physical violence directed at the body and the spirit. In our interviews, we heard many accounts of beatings by police and security guards, particularly the guards who work at one of the major downtown hospitals: "Those five burly security guards horizontally carried me out of [the hospital]—in front of everybody, talk about dignity—put me in the [parking lot]. And five of them look at me . . . and they said, 'Don't you fucking come back here again.' And wham, right in the face." (After we had finished collecting data for this study, assaults committed by hospital security guards in Toronto—particularly against Aboriginal patients and visitors—began to be reported by local media and, for a short while, were a scandal [CBC News 2009a, 2009b, 2009c].) One man experienced his forced psychiatric treatment as assault: "As soon as I was taken to the hospital, I was given a heavy-duty psychotropic drug and then strapped down to a bed for twenty-four hours. I mean, if you weren't psychotic going in, you're definitely psychotic once you're in there. You know? It's not dignified, being strapped to a bed and injected with psychotropic drugs, rather than addressing the real problems in our society that are causing people to flip out on the streets." A psychiatrist reported that her dignity was injured when an agitated patient threw her against a wall.

Finally, there is the social process of *abjection*, when people are made to humble themselves by compromising closely held beliefs or by being forced to associate with material or practices they consider unclean.

Faith-based service provision organizations proselytize to their clients, requiring attention to the word as a condition of receiving food or shelter. Lacking even the paltry sums that allow access to public toilets, people who are homeless must relieve themselves in public places like alleys, parks, or ATM kiosks. Elderly nursing home residents are left to lie in their own urine and feces. (A former Ontario minister of health ignited a dignity controversy when he told the press he was considering wearing a high-absorbency adult diaper for a day so he could better understand the issues facing the province's long-term care facilities.) In an emergency room, a man who does outreach work with drug users witnessed the treatment of an Aboriginal man he knew from the streets:

> He wet himself. He was really drunk and he wet himself. So this kind of set [the doctor] off. . . . It was a woman there, a nurse.
> . . . As soon as that doctor left the room, she speedily come from behind the counter. She got his pants off. She had him dried up and cleaned up and back on the stretcher before this doctor could come back in. [The man began to "act out."] And this doctor, finally he says, "That's it. I've had it now." . . . He says, "Put your pants on." . . . Made him put his wet pants on—this really jerks me around just, you know, reliving it—made him put those wet pants on, had security come and, and he said, "Get that man outta here." . . . But to this guy, to him, that's a place where he goes to seek help, and to be treated that way and with that lack of dignity, without leaving him any respect, no wonder he's peeing himself when he goes in there.

I have chosen to present the social processes of violation as singular and distinct entities. When people talk about dignity, however, the processes are not so cleanly separable. Dependence and restriction often co-occur. Grouping, labeling, and vilification are intertwined in many situations. Suspicion, discrimination, and exclusion share a quality of invidious distinction. There are patterns of clustered violation processes that together form a number of common scenarios—accounts of dignity violation Andrew, Vanessa, and I heard over and over again. One example is *unjust accusation*; another is *reduced circumstances*. A third pattern, although it is configured somewhat differently from the other two, may be described as the *dignity trap*.

In unjust accusation, or what several people called "being centered out," an individual faces an accusation that he or she adamantly insists is untrue. The accusation is made publicly, and the nature of the charge, combined with it being public knowledge, starts a cascade of harms to the individual's dignity. The story with which I began this chapter is one of how an unjust accusation of selling his prescription drugs was eroding a man's dignity. Similar scenarios were recounted time and again in our interviews: A man's small car was buffeted by a truck's slipstream on a narrow, hilly road, leading to a careless driving charge and the loss of his ability to pursue a career as a professional driver. A woman's neighbor called child protective services to report her out of malice, triggering several years' worth of involvement with the courts and the police and much stress-induced physical and mental illness. A student was accused of misusing her school's printers (she had printed several hundred pages in error), resulting in a confrontation with the accuser that escalated to the point where threats were made to call security and have her escorted from the building. (In the denouement of the latter account, the woman told me, "I come in early [one day after the incident] and I wrote on the board, 'Photocopy paper is three cents a page. One hundred equals three dollars. Three cents times two hundred equal six dollars. But what is the price of dignity?'")

When I first started hearing these stories, I (from the security and safety of my privileged life) interpreted them as tales of Kafkaesque arbitrariness. I thought the violation lay in the apparent randomness of the accusations. Slowly, however, I realized that the opposite was true: these were in fact the accounts of people who believed they had been "centered out" not randomly, but "targeted" deliberately and with malicious intent because of who they were. The accusation was understood as an attack on the very core of their being. In unjust accusations, there are, at least, contempt, intrusion, restriction, trickery, labeling, vilification, suspicion, deprivation, and bullying. Unjust accusation thus violates dignity through multiple social processes, which damage exactly because they are personal.

In reduced circumstances, people experience a loss of dignity that is connected to a transition from a higher socioeconomic situation to a lower one. The dignity with which they are treated changes with shifts in their status—from being housed to becoming homeless, from having work to being unemployed, from being clean to appearing unkempt, from driving a sleek new car to driving an old clunker. Andrew met a man whose life story provides an excellent example of the ways dignity may be adversely affected by reduced circumstances: "Dignity has always been important to me. I always have pride in what I do and anything in life, and I try to always help people in their problems and their life skills and that. . . . I used to be a set-up man in a company, setting up die presses and stuff like that, making over seven hundred dollars a week, and that's after taxes." But then injury and illness intervened: "I busted both legs over fourteen years ago [and developed epilepsy over the last four years], and I had to resort to going on social assistance, and I was, my forms of work was limited . . . and now I'm making like $525 a month after taxes." As a result, his life changed dramatically:

> Now to be set back on a forced income, a fixed income, I have to
> resort to going to places like, you know, food banks, standing in
> lineups, traveling by bus and subway where I used to have my own
> motor vehicle and, you know, share an apartment where I had my
> own apartment because of financial circumstances. . . . But my
> esteem now, since I developed epilepsy, this form of illness, it's, it's
> put me back—not being able to do things that I like, you know, like
> to do in life. You know, participate in like, you know, swimming
> and stuff like that and exercise programs. You are limited to only do
> certain amount of things. You've got limitations. . . . Now I cannot
> go out at nighttime unless there's someone with me. I'm not allowed
> to go swimming alone. I'm not allowed to do any major cooking . . .
> or anything like that or be in areas where, you know, shop areas
> where you can hurt yourself or possibly death. And, I don't know,
> I've lost, I've lost a lot of . . . dignity. Like, you know, where I could
> do things on my own, now I have to depend on someone else to help
> me and aid me and, you know, and stuff like that.

He felt his losses acutely in his relationships with other people:

> My family and myself, there's a big barrier now that I don't get
> invited so much to social events as I used to in the past because
> there's less things to talk about like work-wise and stuff like that.

So, so I actually feel I lost some of my, you know, pride that way
. . . So like where I used to make seven hundred dollars a week and
when we go like to Thanksgiving dinners, sometimes I'd be a topic:
. . . *This guy, he works, he's a workaholic* and this and that. Now they
look at me as like, like his time has gone, you know. And it's not my
time has gone. Like I'm at age of fifty, but I can still work and stuff
like that, and I feel like I lost my dignity that way, in that I can't
achieve anything, you know, more in my life than what, because of,
you know, before, before the disease, right? So I think people on
disability feel, feel a lot that way. Not just me as an individual, a lot
of people feel that way.

Indeed, a woman who had lived through a similar reduction in circumstances, moving to subsidized housing after a divorce and illness
caused her income to drop dramatically, told me, "People are so mean
and they make you feel so bad about, pointing their fingers if you don't
have the, if you don't have this kind of car, if you don't have those kind
of shoes, you know, or if you don't have this kind of shirt. . . . It's hard.
It's hard to live in the system, on the system, within the system and,
and, keeping it going with dignity."

Reduced circumstances violate dignity through diminishment, dependence, restriction, exclusion, and deprivation. The aftermath of such
drastic transitions—for example, the state of relying on social assistance—are likely to bring exposure to other violation processes, such as
condescension, dismissal, disregard, contempt, and intrusion. Particularly damaging for many is the memory of the way things used to be—
the person who used to be. Implicit comparisons to other people, and
an explicit awareness of the distance between then and now, exacerbate
the injury to dignity.

Dignity traps are set when individuals make choices or engage in
behaviors they believe will be dignity promoting, but the choices or behaviors backfire, resulting in dignity violation. The existence of such
traps points out how dignity and dignity violation are not necessarily
completely straightforward, but intricately bound to and delicately balanced around specific situational details. A mental health service provider noted that the clients who are most aware of and vocal about their
rights often end up having their dignity violated because health care

providers perceive them as argumentative and antagonistic and respond defensively. A young woman who grew up with an intellectually disabled sister believes her parents made a mistake in insisting that the sister always be treated as though she were "normal," because now the gap between the sister's expectations and her abilities is so great:

> We didn't openly talk about her difficulties with her. There's a lot of reasons why we didn't, but it makes it very hard, I think, for her now to accept her own difficulties. . . . Her own sense of dignity, I think, is impacted by the fact that even though she's treated with dignity . . . she didn't get to talk about the parts where she does have difficulty, to know how to accept that part, I think . . . [because] we didn't help her find a way to accept that part of herself. It was like, "No, no, you're totally normal." And she's like, "Except that I can't ever drive a car, right?"

Many people spoke to us about using volunteerism as a way to enhance their dignity, but such activities could also become a threat to that dignity. One man told me that he wanted to volunteer at a community health center where he had received services, but knew he couldn't afford the transit fare to get there—something that made him feel even worse about himself. I interviewed a woman who had been spending several hours a week helping out at her local food bank, work that "really fulfilled like something in myself." Recently she had learned that because she was on social assistance, she was eligible to be paid a nominal sum each month for her efforts. Now, she found herself torn. She needed the money, but the thought of accepting it was distressing: "It would take away my dignity, that's what I feel like, 'cause I'm doing it because I'm giving back what I've been getting and there are a lot of people who are in need and it's something I can do and I'm doing something about that. So, and I feel good about that. . . . I think if I get paid for it, like, I don't know, it kind of nullifies the process of my dignity."

For many people we interviewed, drug use was a dignity trap. As one man explained, "You may think you're doing yourself good because you're taking your mind out of one space and putting it in another, but you're not. You're kidding yourself. 'Oh, I'll do this and I'll feel great, yeah.' OK. And then later on, when you find out how much trouble you caused because you did that, how good are you going to feel? Not very good at all." Another man described how, like many men and women we spoke to, he had attempted to use drugs to manage the impact of a series of devastating life events, but ultimately found the strategy ineffective: "The more frequency my drug use is, the less dignified I feel. . . . I'm just running away. I'm hiding from something, you know. . . . Yeah, increase in certain type of drug use and behavior is just less and less my dignity gets. Sometimes I get zonked to close or next to nothing and just like this shell existing, you know what I mean. Almost like a zombie." A third man repeated what the Native elders he had consulted told him: "If you become an alcoholic, you become a junkie. What you do is, you give your dignity away, you know. Nobody's taking it from you. You're throwing it away."

Dignity violation is best understood through starkly practical descriptive detail, which I have attempted to provide in recounting this chapter's long list of violation processes and scenarios. A more abstract conceptual examination identifies the common characteristics of these processes and provides a different perspective. In the remainder of this chapter, I lay out nine such characteristics that together help to elucidate—and also to raise questions about—the phenomenon of dignity violation.

The first characteristic is *source*. Dignity violation may originate in acts—words or deeds such as rude verbal exchanges or the contemptuous throwing of pennies or the blows struck by an angry security guard. Such acts begin with the attitudes and behaviors of persons. Violation also may be traced to events, such as in the stories of individuals whose experience of dignity violation began with an injury, a divorce, the onset of a serious illness, or other notable disruptions. Although these violations also may involve individual acts, there is a sense that the acts are secondary to the triggering event, which is something larger. Dignity violation often is consequent to a broader, all-encompassing set of circumstances—such as poverty or the illegality of drugs—that cannot be traced to a single act or event.

Source also encompasses the idea of *locus of control*. That is, some violations are the result of acts, events, or circumstances that are external to the individual and for which the individual bears no responsibility. In such cases, people talk about having their dignity "taken away." Other violations originate internally. When people speak about "giving up" or "giving away" their own dignity or about "lowering" themselves and thereby losing their dignity, they describe behaviors or attitudes that may be engaged in response to an external act, event, or circumstance, but the dignity-damaging element of the violation is seen to reside in the internally located choice of how to respond.

A dignity violation may be described by several characteristics of *scope*. Dignity is violated by micro-level social processes—the doctor's quick glance at his watch, "sir" as a form of address—and by meso- and macro-level processes, such as organizational rules and procedures, government policies, and the centuries-long history of social exclusion experienced by Aboriginal Canadians. Some violations have the quality of universality. They will be judged to be damaging to dignity in all times and places. Torture, enacted through a combination of vilification, deprivation, assault, and abjection, is one such universal violation. Other violations are very much dependent on the context in which they occur. There is nothing inherently damaging to dignity about calling someone's name in an office waiting room, but when that office is where people go to apply for social assistance and rules of confidentiality are meant to prevail, it becomes a violation. A violation may occur primarily at the individual level; that is, it may take place in a conversation between individuals, be based on individual characteristics, and affect mainly the individuals involved. In most instances, condescension or contempt appear to be individual in their scope. Alternatively, a violation may be collective in nature: discrimination and deprivation are most often both directed at and controlled by collective entities. When the transgender community in Ontario was unable to speak at a hearing on amendments to the human rights code, disregard violated the community's collective dignity. These individual and collective aspects of scope are complicated by the transitive quality of dignity: individual-level violations are often experienced as damaging to collectivities, and vice versa.

Violation has a characteristic of *quantity* and a *temporal* quality. Specifically, dignity violations may be described by their number, their frequency, and their duration. Some violations tend to be singular; others, as in the scenarios I have described, occur in clustered multiples.

People speak of their dignity being "stripped," connoting a single, sudden offense, or of it being "eroded," suggesting an accumulation of injuries over time. Some violations derive their power from the fact that they are both common and frequent, occurring over and over again. The people we interviewed were philosophical about rudeness and did not appear to be overly affected by any single rude act. However, as one woman noted, finding oneself in multiple rude encounters over the course of a day or a week or a month "chips away at you." Similarly, some violations are over quickly—a word, a failure to make eye contact, even a physical blow. Others endure for long periods of time and it is because of their duration that dignity is harmed. Dependence and deprivation, for example, damage dignity when they are no longer experienced as temporary but have become entrenched as a way of life.

Execution is the next characteristic of dignity violation. Some violations come about primarily through omission. Indifference and disregard, for example, represent lacunae in recognition. Most other violations work through commission, requiring that decisions be made and acts performed. Execution may be further described by qualities of *intention* and *attribution*. Some violations are deliberate, clearly based in malice. Many contemptuous acts are designed to send or to reinforce the message that a person has no value. Bullying seeks to render one party powerless so that the other party may become more powerful. In other cases, however, there is no intent to harm. In a hospital setting, intrusion simply may be a byproduct of a need to access a body part or a piece of information in order to diagnose or treat disease. Violations also can be parsed for the quality of attribution. Sometimes, people are sure they know why the violation is occurring—because they are poor, perhaps, or because they have a drug problem. In other situations, however—such as when a stranger is stunningly rude or when an individual is unjustly accused—the reason for the violation remains obscure to the person experiencing it.

Finally, underlying and controlling all these other characteristics, there is *perception*. Source, locus of control, scope, quantity, timing, execution, intention, and attribution are qualities of violation that can be perceived. Dignity violation is constituted by degrees of internal or external awareness and interpretation of these qualities, and moments of perception that determine whether a violation is blatant or subtle. As we have seen, in many instances, the presence of witnesses makes the experience of violation more damaging. Several activists I interviewed argued that violation could only become real, and therefore remediable, if both the violator and the violated had "faces." Dignity violation requires, at a minimum, that the violation process, the violator, the violated, and the consequences of violation be visible. These elements then must be interpreted as implicated in a violation. Violation thus depends not just on the enactment of the social processes of violation, but on the awareness and interpretation of these social processes. That is, a dignity violation requires not just that an act, event, or circumstance occur, but also that the act, event, or circumstance be seen and construed as a violation either by the person or group involved in the act, event, or circumstance or by an individual or collective observer of it. As I will explore later, awareness and interpretation are also social processes.

The processes of violation I have presented in this chapter are consistent with what other close examinations of dignity have found. That is, in empirical research and popular literature devoted to explicating the experience of dignity violation—whether in the general population (Fuller 2003; Mann 1998; Margalit 1996; Sennett 2003), for workers (Brooker 2008; Ehrenreich 2001; Hodson 2001; Rayman 2001), among the old, the sick, and the dying (Chochinov et al. 2002; Feder-Alford 2006; Hughes, Davies, and Gudmundsdottir 2008; Moody 1998; Waskul and van der Riet 2002), or in the lives of people who are extremely poor (Farmer 2005; Hoffman and Coffey 2008; Miller and Keys 2001; Reutter et al. 2009)—violation is constituted by failures to recognize a shared humanity (human dignity), as in the processes of disregard or objectification, and by a myriad of constraints on the expression of that humanity (social dignity), as in the processes of discrimination, exclusion, and deprivation. These failures and constraints are embedded in larger social and historical structures, and they affect not only individual and collective dignity, but also individual and collective health.

CHAPTER 2

THE STRUCTURES
THAT DENY DIGNITY

> *The rebuilding of denied human dignity is brought*
> *about . . . [through] changing the structures that*
> *deny this dignity. Recognizing inner dignity without*
> *transforming the structures that deny it will remain*
> *just so many words.*
> —Juan José Tamayo-Acosta (2003)

The first time I spoke to an audience about dignity violation, it was to the staff of an agency that provides health and social care services to homeless and underhoused individuals in Toronto. Midway through my presentation, a listener dismissed my recounting of the social processes of violation as a detailed but aimless inventory of the ways some people have of "being mean" to other people. (He prefaced his remarks by stating he had little use for research.) "What's the point?" My critic continued, "Telling us all about how people are mean to each other doesn't challenge injustice."

Documenting the processes of dignity violation is important for several reasons. Conceptually, violation provides "empirical content" to dignity (Gewirth 1992, 15). Any number of authors have noted that we see dignity most clearly when it is at risk or once it has been lost: "One of the best approaches to an exploration in depth of what human dignity means is to start from the experience of 'indignation'" (Spiegelberg 1970, 60). We discover dignity "through its opposite" (Dussel 2003, 93). That is, an understanding of dignity violation deepens our understanding of dignity itself. In practice, a comprehensive catalog of violations is crucial to realizing the prescriptive uses of dignity. As Jonathan Mann (1997, 1998) argued, the work of amelioration begins with identifying and describing the many types and permutations of dignity violation; such identification and description can then be applied analytically to explore how social dignity may affect health status and other important dignity outcomes, and the resulting knowledge integrated into policy and practice in order to devise effective interventions. Detailed accounts of dignity violation also can be marshaled to raise moral awareness—to give voice to that which is often experienced, but too rarely articulated. In all these ways, holding the social processes of dignity violation up to the light can be instructive. Indeed, at the same presentation, others were quick to begin a conversation about how an improved understanding of dignity violation might be used to change the ways in which they designed and delivered their services.

Any dignity violation can be broken down into several moving parts: the act, or the process or processes of violation (the subject of Chapter 1); the actors involved; the context; and the consequence. Specific violations can be conceptualized as the outcomes of specific *dignity encounters,* or dignity-laden interactions that take place between specific actors in specific times and places—the context in which the encounter is situated. Analyzing context means examining a number of such encounters singly and together, paying attention to any patterns that emerge in the connections between social processes, actors, context, and consequence. These patterns are the contextual conditions of dignity violation.

There are four main types of contextual conditions: conditions that pertain to the positions of the actors involved in a specific dignity encounter—actors that may include individuals, organizations, geographic communities or communities of affinity, and whole societies; conditions that pertain to the nature of the relationship between the actors; conditions that pertain to the setting in which the encounter takes place; and conditions pertaining to the social order in which actors, encounters, and settings all are situated. These conditions are layered, overlapping. In some instances, they may best be conceptualized as risk factors, features of the encounter that increase the chances that violation will occur. At other times, the conditions are themselves constitutive of violation. The four types of conditions are linked to one another: certain kinds of relationships between actors are more common in certain kinds of settings, for example. While conditions and violation processes tend to be patterned, the possibility of dignity promotion (which I explore conceptually in Chapter 4 and again, more practically, in Chapter 5) suggests that no single condition or set of conditions need always be determinative of violation and, further, that conditions themselves are mutable.

Dignity violation is facilitated when an (individual or collective) actor in a dignity encounter is in a *position of vulnerability*. Vulnerability may be conferred internally or externally, by physical, psychological, or social attributes. The word "position" is important here, because it indicates that the state of being vulnerable is not necessarily inherent, nor is it unalterable. Rather, vulnerability is contingent.

Actors become vulnerable to dignity violation in demanding situations. One such situation is the phenomenon of the life transition. The transition from comfort to poverty, the scenario of reduced circumstances described in Chapter 1, is an example. In interviews, people spoke of other transitions—disjunctions or turning points—that made them vulnerable: when they were beginning or ending a romantic relationship, when they were faced with a change to their parental status (such as a threatened loss of custody), when they were learning to live with a chronic illness, or when they were growing old.

A second such situation is crisis, periods of instability or turmoil. A man who provides support to people with mental health problems described the vulnerability occasioned by the cascades of personal and financial emergencies experienced by his clients:

> Especially for some clients who have just had a major life change,
> lost a job, you know, lost family support, or have just been diagnosed
> with a mental illness or some other illness and are really struggling
> to get their lives, you know, on track. . . . Trying to scrape by, with
> no money, living in poverty, living with no money, living with
> no food or, you know, worrying about your next meal, worrying
> about where you're going to stay. It's hard to find dignity in those
> situations, you know?

Vulnerability closely follows need. Both absolute and relative deprivation violate dignity, in part by putting people in a position of being needy. When asked in what situations he thought people were at greatest risk of dignity violation, one man I interviewed replied, as though it should be obvious, "People living where they require the help." In such situations, the man whose experience of reduced circumstances I described in Chapter 1 said, "You feel some of your pride is gone. Like, you know, you feel you're lowering yourself going to places [e.g., food banks] where you thought you'd never, you know, ever end up and, you know, places like that." Being needy is shameful, and shame, another man told us, is also a position of vulnerability, one that works by making people "just feel like they're worthless and useless." The shame that follows deprivation and its common sequela of exposure to indifference, dismissal, and diminishment thus leaves people vulnerable to future dignity violations.

Being different is another position of vulnerability. Both of the transgender women we interviewed spoke of the ways in which their visible physical differences ("Oh, he's a man with really big breasts") made them vulnerable to insult and injury. Members of minority racial or ethnic groups described how their differences from "mainstream Canadians" seemed to provoke heightened scrutiny, such as in their interactions with shopkeepers, and physical violence, such as in their encounters with police. A Black man whose working-class family had lived in a "very wealthy Northern European" neighborhood in one of the Maritime provinces for more than a century told Vanessa a story of how his differences led to verbal abuse and social exclusion: "The kids called me a nigger, because they said their mommy 'told me don't talk to that nigger' . . . so I was constantly called names. . . . At the same time, I'm told to get out of my, get out of someone's country and go back to Africa and swing from the trees like a monkey. . . . Even my teachers in school called me names." His differences were exacerbated, and his dignity further affronted, when he began to have problems at home and ended up a ward of the state:

> Every second Friday from ages nine until twelve, so [grades] four,
> five, and six, a big black car would come up to [the school], the rich
> school, eh? And I had to leave an hour early, so the kids knew . . .
> the child welfare services were making me go to a psychiatrist . . .
> and they'd get the black car to pick me up at the school. . . . And

it's bad if I was the only person of color [at the school], but then it's also getting picked up—no one else gets picked up in a big black car, mysterious-like.

Mental illness and drug addiction place people in vulnerable positions in a number of ways. First, several people we spoke to described how symptoms of mental disorders or the effects of craving or taking drugs may lead to conduct that is less than dignified. A mental health service provider spoke of seeing in her clients "shame and embarrassment around behaviors that people engaged in while unwell . . . challenges with their decision-making or their judgment." A number of people who had struggled with drugs told us that drugs had "taken away [their] humanness" because of the acts they had committed while high or seeking a high.

Second, mental illness and addiction labels often lead people to be discredited. Once "you say you have a mental illness," one woman noted, [other people] "automatically assume a lot of things about you that may or may not be true." She described "the stigma that's attached [to] people because of . . . what they're thought of." (One man called this phenomenon of discredit "that mental health frigging trap.") Similarly, another woman told us, being an addict brings with it the assumption that "you're a useless hunk of flesh."

Vulnerability also attaches to the circumstances in which people may find themselves when they are experiencing mental illness or addiction. Individuals we interviewed who had been hospitalized in psychiatric facilities described how upon admission their "dignity went from sixty to zero in like two minutes flat" through processes of diminishment, intrusion, and restriction. The very first thing the mental health system does, one man told me, "it says, we think you're no good." The risk of violation is also high in the community, where people who have been addicted to illicit drugs or suffered from mental illness for a long time without receiving adequate support often will find themselves caught in what a mental health service provider described as a "downward social drift . . . into poverty, you know, sort of penury and, and homelessness and that sort of thing."

Transition, crisis, need, difference, and mental illness and addiction are examples of positions of vulnerability, but that list is by no means exhaustive. In our interviews, and in the literature, physical illness, pain, old age, low levels of education, physical or psychological weakness, timidity, voicelessness, invisibility, fear, and anger were also identified as states that make actors vulnerable to dignity violation. As with the processes of dignity violation, these states seem to cluster, to co-occur either concurrently or sequentially. Particular vulnerabilities or patterns of vulnerability may be linked to certain processes of violation. Abjection may be experienced both by aged individuals who wear diapers because they are physically unable to use a toilet without help and by homeless and destitute younger people who cannot afford the dollar that buys a coffee and access to the toilet that is "for customers only." The sharp-eyed reader will have noticed that in addition to conferring vulnerability to dignity violation, many of these positions may also be the result of dignity violation. In this way, often through the microprocesses I will explore later in this chapter, dignity violation may become self-perpetuating.

In dignity encounters that result in violation, one also finds actors who are in a *position of antipathy*, a state of aversion or opposition to the other actors in the encounter. There are different kinds and degrees of antipathy, as demonstrated in a range of attitudes and behaviors; these different forms seem to be associated with different processes of violation. As with vulnerability, antipathy is not necessarily a fixed position. Rather, it is shaped by other conditions in the encounter.

One man related a vivid story of a methadone clinic receptionist with what he called a "make-wrong attitude," or "an analytical computation the individual uses to make themself right by making others wrong." In this particular incident, the man arrived at the clinic about ten minutes before closing. The receptionist was busy with another client and told him to wait. He had to urinate, and because the clinic did not have a toilet available for client use, asked if he could leave to do so:

> And they told me to go ahead and come back, and then I wasn't there, I wasn't there [at closing time.] And it wasn't as if . . . [they] didn't know. I was just there. They knew I didn't have my [dose]. They knew I was coming back, and they chose not to [wait]. . . . I'm talking to her the next day, and it's like she's making me wrong . . . it's my responsibility to see that I am there before [closing]. Well,

you couldn't wait five minutes, you know? So how do you justify putting me into withdrawal for the sake of five minutes when you told me to go ahead and come back when you knew I had to find a washroom. . . . Why would you say "go ahead" and then, having said that, lock the doors and leave, you know, before I came back to get my methadone?

The people we interviewed often described their interactions with low-level government employees in ways that emphasized the antipathy they sensed the workers held toward their jobs and their clients. One woman talked about her probation officer: "And then I got to report to some jerk, pardon my language, but he's from another country, which is fine, but I can't quite understand him. He's younger than me, and he's got a chip on his shoulder bigger than I don't know." A man reported his experience with social assistance workers:

They're really bad for taking your dignity away. . . . I mean, when you go in there and you ask for their help . . . first, they're grumpy. I don't know why. You go in there to get help. "Fill this out." "Wait here. Wait there" [spoken in a gruff voice]. It's not, "Sir, you have to go over here and wait" [spoken in a pleasant voice]. . . . And they make, like within five minutes, they make you feel like you shouldn't be there.

A woman who also had received social assistance observed that any worker "who's been in that system, in the disability system for over five or ten years . . . they get calloused. . . . It just gets to the point where they're nonfeeling. It's just like, you know, the cow coming in for the slaughter, you know. Just, we're all the same, just process us, just cover our asses, just make sure everything, all the i's are dotted and get us the hell out of there." A social worker who provides services to homeless individuals concurred, noting that many welfare office employees seem to think of clients "as a waste of their time and in many ways will tell you that."

Other antipathies are demonstrated by arrogance—what a man described to us as a sense people have that "they are socially superior, better off than you are, and so they can . . . out-snob anybody." The men and women we interviewed often found such antipathy in doctors and other high-status professionals. One man used the word "complacent" to describe many of the physicians he had met. He noted: "Sometimes I think people get a big head on them, you know, 'cause they're doctors and, and sure they have a lot of knowledge. . . . I'm not negating that, but I think people should realize that the learning process doesn't stop. There's things you can learn off, off of everybody." A legal aid lawyer reported that in the adversarial environment of the courtroom, she sometimes saw her colleagues attempt to "humiliate" and "break down" opposing parties, thus demonstrating their own arrogant antipathy:

> One of the worst things that lawyers did . . . [was to say of an underemployed client, in open court,] "Why can't he get a better job? He's got all this time on his hands." That's harsh, you know? Especially since we've already obviously put down on paper all the reasons why somebody can't get a better job or pay more. . . . I had a lawyer come up to my client—which they aren't supposed to do, they're supposed to talk to me—and say, "You look like a strapping young lad," or ,"You look like you can work, how come you're not working? How come you can't get a job? What's wrong with you?"

"The higher you go," another woman told me, "the smaller the 'd' in dignity."

For the people we interviewed, the worst sort of antipathy was represented by what a woman described as the "human predators" who "aggressively chew on your true feeling [about] yourself and take away your dignity . . . because they sense your weakness." One man had observed such a tendency toward predation in some detox counselors:

> The most treacherous are the ones that are themselves recovering alcoholics or they identify themselves as recovering alcoholics. So in the detoxes it's pretty well counselors that are dealing with their own alcoholism. And then it becomes a kind of a, this waltz. Something cruel about it. They do things like withholding information they know would be of value to certain clients that want to get out of the system. And they can sometimes keep you locked in longer than you need to be there. But because of your own

vulnerability at the time, you're just not thinking right. You're not thinking with clarity, you know? You lose that dignity and become compliant and meek.

"Power-tripping" police and security guards also demonstrate this kind of antipathy. One man said of the police, "You feel like a real criminal when they get you, you know? They, they sometimes they beat you, when you're trying to tell them your side, your statement or whatever, like they don't believe you, you know, or something, you know? They just, I don't know, it's like they have lots of anger or something or you've, it's like you made them do some work or something, right, them having to arrest you."

These examples are, again, meant to be illustrative, not comprehensive. In our interviews, actors who are self-serving, self-absorbed, jealous, stupid, incompetent, or impatient are also seen to be in positions of antipathy. What the examples I have presented suggest is that antipathy may manifest in different ways, leading to different processes of violation. The grumpiness of the social service bureaucrat is associated with rudeness and indifference; the arrogance of the professional with condescension and trickery; the viciousness of the predator with bullying and assault. As antipathy grows more extreme, the other actors in an encounter are more likely to be seen as something less than human. As perceived humanness diminishes, the way is paved for the enactment of more and more severe—more universally recognized, more collective, more numerous, more frequent, more enduring, more deliberate—processes of dignity violation.

Earlier, I noted the significance of the language of position and the fact that neither vulnerability nor antipathy are fixed. Indeed, any actor may find himself in either of these positions. As some of the quotations I have used suggest, antipathy often begets antipathy. (The reader might wonder just who stands in a position of antipathy when a woman refers to her probation officer as a "jerk" and feels compelled to emphasize the fact that he is an immigrant.) The actor who is in a position of vulnerability may step into a position of antipathy, and vice versa. When I was interviewing health and social service providers, I asked what made it difficult for them to treat their clients with dignity. They often responded by describing times when they themselves became vulnerable—perhaps when a client grew physically violent—or when their clients demonstrated obvious antipathy toward them—for example, when a client used abusive or personally offensive language.

Movement between positions of vulnerability and antipathy is possible because of the highly relational quality of dignity encounters. Actors play off one another, and the nature of their interactions is shaped not just by the positions they hold individually, but also by the nature of the connections between them. In general, dignity violation is more frequent in encounters where the relationship between the actors is characterized by *asymmetry*. Not all facets of the relationship need be asymmetrical for the threat of violation to materialize. However, asymmetry in the dimensions that are important to the particular encounter seems to increase the likelihood of violation.

In health care, dignity encounters are often characterized by intertwined asymmetries of information or knowledge and power or authority between the actors. Actors in positions of vulnerability are acutely aware of these asymmetries:

> I had an appointment a week ago and it was a new doctor . . . and he was taking a while . . . which I understand because he was new to my case. But I asked him, "Is there something that's concerning you right now?" And he said, "Oh, no! Nothing's wrong! Nothing's wrong!" And he was in a rush to leave the room and discuss whatever was on his mind with the [other] doctor rather than just saying to me there might be, you know, something I'm concerned about. . . . But he didn't want to tell me anything and he didn't want, you know, to answer my question truthfully.

A woman whose nurse dismissed her complaints about what turned out to be a very serious postsurgical complication ("Well, you need to accept that you just had surgery and that you're going to be in pain") said, "This [nurse] is going to do nothing for me. Because she is too much into this what I call crazy behavior that I see some people get into. If they've got power over you, they do something crazy. . . . They abuse it. I was helpless." Another woman described all patients as being in a "one down" position in interactions with their health care providers: "They are in a—they're either frightened or helpless or ignorant—very much in a one down position as a result, because they are seeking the help of an expert." In psychiatric hospitals, a man explained, asymmetry stands as a barrier to people helping themselves:

> If you have no power, how are you going to have the toolkit to recover your dignity? If you have no understanding of what they're doing, how do you have the toolkit to communicate with the people in order to find out how to get out of the situation you're in or even explain the situation you're in? So without knowledge and without a parity of, of communication or an equal social standing with a health care professional, which is not possible when you're under their care anyway, you're hung out to dry.

I was struck in the stories we heard by how infrequently people seemed to confront their health care providers directly or to make formal complaints about even the most egregious ill treatment in hospitals and other medical facilities. As one woman said, "Other people that I would encounter on a daily basis, I wouldn't let them treat me that way." When I asked about people's reluctance to lodge grievances or even just to make known their displeasure, the same woman told me: "They're the people who have more authority over you to make you feel that way. . . . I let them do it. Maybe. But maybe I feel it's because they're in a position of higher up that I have to take this. I really don't. But, really, you do." And a man said, "You're afraid to go against a doctor, like going against a lawyer or God. Like, you know, they got money and power." In part, people hesitated to "go against" their health care providers because they foresaw ending up in confrontations in which credibility would also be asymmetrical (in the health care professional's favor). One woman explained why she had declined to lodge complaints against hospital personnel even after several incidents of very poor care:

> I would probably report things more often if I knew that my word would be taken as seriously as the word of the staff. There's nothing worse than raising a complaint and then finding out later that the staff person said, "Oh, that didn't happen." And then all of a sudden

if they say it didn't happen, then it didn't happen. Or it didn't happen the way you said it did. You're embellishing or you're what not.

Several people described staying silent because they feared retaliation in the form of a denial of future care. Doctors, in particular, one person told me, "have the power to provide or withhold particular services, particular letters of referral, particular opportunities."

The same asymmetries, and some new ones, occur in other kinds of dignity encounters. In the offices where decisions are made about eligibility for social assistance, workers have the power to deny applicants access to money and other desperately needed resources. In almost all types of social care, there is an imbalance of personal information: the provider will know many intimate details about the life of the client, while the client will know very little about the provider. As one social worker told me, this asymmetry leads people to feel "at my mercy in some way . . . that I'll talk about them to someone or that I'll laugh at them or . . . that I'll somehow use the information against them."

Unlike position, asymmetry is not so easily changed. Qualities like wealth or knowledge will not suddenly shift in favor of one actor from another during a dignity encounter. What may change, however, are the terms of the encounter, the dimensions of the relationship that are the most important. In the following incident, a client in a "one down" position, whose dignity had been injured because of a provider's exercise of professional power, attempted to overturn the asymmetry by using a threat of violence:

I needed to get a letter for [the mental health court] from my worker . . . stating that borderline personality disorder contributes to shoplifting, and it does. It's one of the nine criteria. And I also, you know, made sure that I wasn't using this as an excuse . . . but I got a problem. So if you can just put that in writing, give it to the [mental health court] worker, we can get this going. What did she say to me? "No, I won't write you a letter because I want you to, you know, take responsibility for what you've done, and I want you to hang out with poor people so that you can get a better appreciation of what it means to have people who are less fortunate than you so that you'll stop shoplifting." And I hang out with poor people and severely mentally ill people who are poorer than me already. What, you know. So that was, that was, that was going beyond her boundaries. So eventually I said [to a colleague of the provider who had refused to write the letter], "Well, if I don't get this letter from her I'm going to kill her."

(In this rather extreme example, the attempt to revise the terms of the encounter by changing which kind of power would be most important in the relationship became a dignity trap: the threat did not persuade the provider to produce a letter, but it did result in the client being violently apprehended by the police and ultimately going to prison.)

All dignity encounters unfold in specific physical and social environments, settings that host both the actors and their actions and interactions. Settings may be conceptualized as geographic locations, like street corners; they may be organizations or institutions, like the offices of a service provision agency or a hospital; they may be larger sociopolitical units, like a city. Settings also may be more abstract entities—the emotional and psychological spaces that are created by families, for example. The settings in which dignity violation is most likely to occur seem to be characterized by *harsh circumstances*. That is, they are physical and social places and spaces in which customary boundaries (such as those of aesthetics, hygiene, modesty, or privacy) are often transgressed, disorder reigns, resources are scarce, people are stressed and distracted, emotions run high, and rules are seemingly both uneven and unyielding.

A number of people we spoke to described their earliest experiences of dignity violation as taking place in their families. One man recollected his relationship with his brothers: "My brothers were all the time criticizing me and putting me down, you know, all the time. I've always had that, especially with my younger brother. . . . My younger brothers, two of them, one of them in particular, was all the time criticizing me, heckling me, putting me down. And I never liked that. That sort of took away a sense of my pride and my dignity." Another woman talked about the roots of her own shaky dignity in her family environment: "I grew up in a really violent home life, and you know you rarely find physical abuse without emotional . . . so I'm not sure which, it's probably the combination of the both. You always feel as though you're not up to par . . . you're not up to par, the sky's going to fall at any minute. And anytime something did happen, you better watch your back 'cause it's going to get bad, right?"

For many of the people we spoke to, their homes continued to be settings for dignity violation. Several women who were living in subsidized housing described the ways in which housing complex residents (most often other women) sniped at, competed with, and scapegoated one another. Everyone in her building was poor, one woman told me, and "a lot of the people have mental illness, and yet they all stigmatize other people, even though—it's like because, well, I've had it done to me, so I'm going to do it to you. It's horrendous."

A similar dynamic seems to exist in homeless shelters, which are meant for short-term accommodation, but where some people live for months at a time. The regimentation of daily life in the shelters, the crowding, and the filth, combined with the stresses of the social services "runaround," create high-pressure environments that are dangerous to dignity. One man described shelters as places where one is told "when to go to sleep, when to eat. . . . I would prefer to be broke sleeping in the snow bank, honestly. . . . Because of the fact that it takes away everything that you, not you, you're a number to them, and as a number, they can do anything. No, that's very stressful and zero dignity and strung [out]. You are stressed. . . . One hour seems like a day in there." Another man agreed, telling me, "Nobody really wants to [sleep on the street] but many people choose that over a shelter or rooming house." I asked him why that was. "Well, for me, it was because of the, the threat of violence, the proliferation of hard drugs, the vermin and disease, bedbugs."

I have written about how health care settings, particularly large institutions, tend to be chronically short of space, equipment and materials, and time (Jacobson 2009b) and thus often are dangerous to dignity. As one man observed about his hospitalization experience, "I think a lot of the nursing staff and other caregivers are way overtaxed." The asymmetrical relations between providers and patients (as well as the asymmetries of status and authority between professional groups, such as those between physicians and nurses) contribute to an atmosphere of fear, hostility, and rigidity. The circumstances that bring people into these settings tend to be sources of great anxiety, which also work to put people in positions of vulnerability. Hospital emergency departments might be the quintessential cases of all these elements combined. (Elements that are compounded by sleeplessness and fatigue: a number of people noted that dignity was at greater risk on the night shift.) Indeed, in our interviews, we heard over and over again how indifference, dismissal, intrusion, discrimination, exclusion, and even assault (as I have noted, most often by hospital security guards) and abjection were common experiences in ERs.

The city of Toronto provides an example of how a larger-scale sociopolitical entity may manifest the kinds of harsh circumstances that are associated with dignity violation (Jacobson, Oliver, and Koch 2009). The Torontonians we interviewed talked about how environmental characteristics of the city structured the processes of violation they had experienced. Among the conditions they cited were inconvenient location of social services and other resources, expensive (and sometimes exclusionary) public transit, bad weather, a shortage of affordable housing, poorly constructed buildings, noise, dirt, and the scarcity of public toilets. In addition, many people described how the average city dweller's public façade of hurry, preoccupation, and toughness created an atmosphere that was frantic and uncaring, and thus threatening to dignity.

At the most encompassing level of context, dignity violation is associated with a *social order of inequality*. The men and women we interviewed often reflected on the ways in which the dignity violations they had experienced could, in the final analysis, be attributed to broad societal structures of inequity, such as entrenched poverty or racism, and to the collective attitudes and practices that promote and maintain these structures.

The people we spoke to who were poor and who had experienced the kinds of violations associated with need often looked beyond their own particular circumstances to point out how the insults and injuries to their dignity were part of a larger problem, a "bigotry of the haves against the have-nots." Such bigotry was demonstrated through messages that the poor were responsible for their own poverty—"just a bunch of no goods that, that could have it good in this world and in this country because we have such a great strong economy"—and a corresponding unwillingness to ameliorate poverty by increasing the minimum wage or funding social assistance programs adequately. Several of the interview participants who identified themselves as political activists took the point further, attributing this bigotry to a culture in which the highest value is materialism and to the power of corporations to shape such cultural values and thus dictate the terms of the social contract. They also described how economically powerful groups manipulated those on the margins to set them against each other, establishing a "hierarchy of oppression" that "plays itself out in oppressed groups" and dilutes the ability of these groups to work together for societal change. "The way our system is set up," one man told me, "it's very hard for anyone below the poverty line to fight for their rights."

Similarly, people who had experienced dignity violations that they believed were linked to racial or ethnic status saw the actions and attitudes of the individuals they encountered as indicative of societal-level conditions. An African immigrant, a man who endured a series of dignity violations during a lengthy period of involvement with the justice system, eventually reached the conclusion that the system itself was "manufacturing criminals" and that racial prejudice, while not the only factor in who was criminalized, made criminalization a more likely outcome. An Aboriginal man argued that police could be brutal to anyone, but that widely held stereotypes of his people lent him a particular kind of vulnerability to such brutality: "Because I'm Native, they look even worse on me. . . . They accuse you because you're Native, say you're a drunk, your family is a drunk or stuff like that."

The social order as perceived by many of the people we interviewed was deeply unfair. Vanessa spoke to a woman who told her matter-of-factly, "There's two laws: there's laws for you and there's laws for us. . . . They treat you with respect. They treat you with dignity. They would not *not* believe you." Vanessa asked, "And then for you, when you deal with them, what does it look like?" "Automatically not believed," the woman answered. "I'm like, I'm just a piece of garbage." The African immigrant said, "We're still living in a world where we are not together. We still are separate. There's a lot of, a lot of walls separates people." According to one woman, such inequities and divisions are erected and maintained by what she called "9/11 thinking," a pervasive paranoia, distrust, and fear exploited by corporations and governments that want "to keep us scared and . . . to keep [our] dignity at bay."

Confirmation of the importance of these conditions—positions of vulnerability and antipathy, asymmetry, harsh circumstances, and a social order of inequality—to collective, as well as individual, dignity violation may be found in a wide array of literature that describes the phenomenon of violation in a number of different arenas. In workplaces, we see that those most prone to dignity violation are low-wage, low-skill workers whose employment is precarious (Brooker 2008; Ehrenreich 2001). According to Barbara Ehrenreich (2001), the antipathy of midlevel managers toward these workers is the defining characteristic of minimum-wage businesses like retail operations or cleaning companies: "For reasons that have more to do with class—and often racial—prejudice than with actual experience, [supervisory personnel] tend to fear and distrust the category of people from which they recruit their workers. Hence the perceived need for repressive management and intrusive measures like drug and personality testing" (212). Asymmetries of authority are built into the structure of most workplaces, but settings in which management wields unilateral power have been shown to be more destructive to workers' dignity (Hodson 2001). Similarly, workplaces that manifest harsh circumstances like chronic disorganization and mismanagement, overwork, and underpayment also see more violations of dignity (ibid.; Rayman 2001). Of course, overwork and underpayment are more likely to be valorized in a "bottom line culture" (Rayman 2001, 37) that values profit over all else.

Erving Goffman's *Asylums* (1961), the classic study of life in a psychiatric hospital, focuses on the social processes of dignity violation in such total institutions and reveals some of the same conditional patterns. Goffman recounts in minute detail how hospitalization sets off for the "recruit," already vulnerable by virtue of whatever events have brought him to the hospital, "a series of abasements, degradations, humiliations, and profanations of self. His self is systematically, if often unintentionally, mortified" (14). The mortification is reinforced by staff attitudes and behaviors that demonstrate antipathy toward the recruit (justified as necessary in order to compel him to recognize and accept his sickness) and by the asymmetries of information, communication, and control between inmates and their keepers. The dignity-violating practices of the asylum reflect a social order that disdains and fears people who are labeled as mentally ill.

Bureaucratic responses to poverty, like homelessness relief and social assistance, already identified by the men and women we interviewed as some of the prime sites for dignity violation, also involve many of these conditions. Lisa Hoffman and Brian Coffey (2008) argue that the dignity-denying environment of many homeless shelters is a result of chronic underfunding and service fragmentation, which cause chaos and stress for shelter clients and staff alike. In their comparative study of welfare systems in four countries, Chak Kwan Chan and Graham Bowpitt (2005) show how the dignity-denying elements of these systems reflect broader features of the countries' national ideologies and political economies: "Hong Kong's free market welfare system attempts to safeguard its low tax and limited labour protection system by reinvigorating the work ethic and enhancing personal and family responsibilities. As a result, the self-esteem and social respect of [welfare recipients] have been undermined" (63).

Antipathies and asymmetries between social care workers and recipients are exacerbated in relationships that are one-off rather than sustained. Among the changes to the Ontario's disability support system made by a Conservative government in the 1990s was a decree that offices shift to a "team" style of case management, thus ensuring that workers and clients would have very little opportunity to develop the kind of familiarity that enhances human connection (*Barriers to ODSP* 2003). One Toronto activist I interviewed remembered a time when "you could even have a worker come to you . . . to help people with their difficulties." With the policy change, however, the province "cut all that out, 'cause I think there was attachments and workers would go beyond the call to ensure that people got their basic needs met, right?" Now, "that's pretty much gone and [you've got] a lot of new baby workers with very little understanding and, uh, you know, the myths [and stereotypes] about people who are collecting benefits are vast." More broadly, in most welfare societies the relationship between taxpayers and social assistance recipients is characterized by implicit asymmetries—such as those of pity and expectations of gratitude—that heighten the humiliations attendant upon receiving aid (Margalit 1996).

Modern slavery, as described by antislavery activist Kevin Bales (2007), is constituted by a set of dignity violations that includes trickery, exploitation, bullying, assault, and abjection. Those forced into slavery are often women and children, groups made vulnerable because they lack status and power in their households and communities. Bales argues that the slave trade, while driven by greed, is underpinned by prejudice and bigotry, historical collective antipathies based on race, ethnicity, and caste. Its continued existence is supported by the harsh circumstances of widespread desperation and corruption linked to poverty, sentinels of a social order that is deeply inequitable.

The narratives of people we interviewed and these examples drawn from the literature suggest that each contextual condition is closely linked to the other conditions. Conditions resonate with one another and amplify each other's effects. Being in a position of vulnerability makes harsh circumstances all the more difficult to bear. One actor's antipathy may exacerbate another actor's vulnerability. Linkages between conditions may be temporal. Present conditions are often the result of past conditions. Repeated experiences of harsh circumstances in the past predispose people to positions of antipathy in the present. Conditions may relate to one another like matryoshkas, the collections of wooden Russian dolls in which the smaller are contained by the larger. Broad conditions, such as social order, determine narrower conditions, such as the asymmetries between actors that may be identified in particular dignity encounters.

Contextual conditions are intertwined with the social processes of violation and their characteristics. Specific vulnerabilities and antipathies may be associated with specific processes of violation or with specific clusters of these processes. Past processes of violation create present conditions—just as present conditions will help to create future processes of violation. The characteristics of violation—source, locus of control, scope, quantity, timing, execution, intention, attribution, and perception—are also structured by conditions. Violation processes situated primarily in positions of antipathy may be more particular and individual in scope, while those situated primarily in a social order of inequality may be more universal and collective. Violations associated with a setting's harsh circumstances are more likely to be perceived as inadvertent acts of omission, while those based on an individual's particular position of vulnerability may be interpreted as deliberate acts of commission.

I said earlier that conditions may be viewed both as risk factors for violation and as constitutive of violation in and of themselves. Conditions are risk factors when they put people in situations that increase the chances of violation. Being needy means a person will be more likely to find herself in places like food banks or welfare offices where dignity violation is common. Interacting with an actor who is in a position of antipathy increases the odds that a dignity encounter will be destructive. Asymmetry facilitates social processes like condescension and dependence. Another way of saying this is that conditions may operate as threats to dignity—threats that may or may not be realized. Conditions constitute violation when they not only structure the social processes of violation but also actually enact these processes. Many of the qualities that describe harsh circumstances are dignity violations in and of themselves. A social order of inequality is built on a multitude of individual and collective asymmetries, such as those of wealth, privilege, and political power. Whether a condition is seen as a risk factor or as a violation is in part a matter of perspective.

In a sense, the entire notion of the dignity encounter may be an artifact, a construction of method and analysis. We began each interview by asking our participants to describe "a time when dignity was important to you." Many people, as I have already noted, came to the interviews with a particular act or event or circumstance they wanted to discuss and were easily prompted by this question. Others, however, resisted our framing, arguing that dignity was "important all the time." This response suggests that dignity cannot always be located in a specific time or place. It is neither created nor destroyed through particular actions or interactions, because dignity in the present is bound to the past and the future. One also can question the conditions I have described. Indeed, they, and the individual social processes of violation, may be seen not as separate and distinct phenomena, but as the same phenomenon viewed from different perspectives or at different levels of focus. For the critic I introduced at the beginning of this chapter—the listener who was scornful of my description of the social processes of violation—both what happened in a micro-level dignity encounter between individual actors and the meso-level conditions that might structure this kind of encounter were irrelevant, because the only condition of any consequence was the inequitable social order.

The social processes of violation—rudeness, indifference, condescension, dismissal, diminishment, disregard, dependence, restriction, objectification, intrusion, contempt, trickery, grouping, labeling, vilification, suspicion, discrimination, exclusion, exploitation, revulsion, deprivation, bullying, assault, and abjection—are mediated through the mechanisms of awareness and interpretation, the characteristic of perception I introduced at the end of Chapter 1. It is through these microprocesses that dignity violation is recognized and acknowledged. To understand awareness and interpretation—to understand what is happening inside, or underneath, the social processes of violation—we return to the dignity encounter. In such an encounter, the actors involved—including those individual or collective actors who may be witnessing the encounter—engage in a series of reciprocal actions, including reading markers, making gestures, interpreting these markers and gestures, and responding to them. Because the process is cyclical, it cannot be said to begin or end at any particular point. However, for ease of explication, I will begin with the dignity marker.

Dignity markers are closely related, although not identical, to Goffman's widely used concept of stigma, "a special discrepancy between virtual and actual social identity . . . an attribute that is deeply discrediting" (1963, 3): "First, there are abominations of the body—the various physical deformities. Next there are blemishes of individual character perceived as weak will, domineering or unnatural passion, treacherous and rigid beliefs, and dishonesty. . . . Finally, there are the tribal stigma of race, nation, and religion" (4). Like stigma, dignity markers are "signs that convey social information" about the "more or less abiding characteristics" of an individual (43). "The information, as well as the sign through which it is conveyed, is reflexive and embodied" (43). Dignity markers thus are a set of sensory, most often visual, cues that indicate whether or not the bearer "has" dignity, and thus whether or not this actor "deserves" to be treated with dignity. They are either part of the body or otherwise attached to the person (for example, as a coded notation in an individual's medical record). While some markers can be hidden, others cannot easily be concealed. Both individual and collective actors display dignity markers.

Through social comparison, actors are highly attuned to the significance of these markers. In our interviews, people spoke of things like dress, personal possessions, cleanliness, and even telephone numbers as dignity markers. In North America, dentition is a very powerful marker:

> I didn't have bottom teeth. Like I had teeth, but I didn't have the plate. I had lost it when I was drunk. [The speaker had called his brother to ask for money to replace the dental plate, but his brother refused to provide it.] And I was totally devastated. [The speaker had to make a court appearance on a serious charge.] It wasn't a joke. I didn't find it a joke. . . . I said, "What's wrong with you? Are you nuts? You think I wanna stand there in court and look like that?"

The men and women we interviewed often rejected the idea that the dignity violations they had experienced were somehow provoked by their own behavior. However, they did acknowledge that these violations were linked to their deeply held feelings of inadequacy or inferiority—psychological states that they believed could be perceived by others. One woman told me how physical demeanor—in particular, a hunched-over posture she described as demonstrating a state of "being wounded"—served as a dignity marker and could leave people vulnerable to violation.

Respect (and by extension, disrespect) is an "expressive performance" (Sennett 2003, 207). Gestures are the communicative acts through which respect and disrespect are performed. Spoken language is a gesture—both in the form of specific words (addressing a transgender woman as "sir" or an African Canadian boy as "nigger") and tone of voice (a nurse using a "singsong" tone to speak to an adult patient). So too is body language. According to the men and women we interviewed, some of the nonverbal gestures that convey disrespect include not looking directly at an actor who is speaking, staring when an actor is seeking modesty, flinching when physical contact is made or ostentatiously avoiding such contact, eye rolling, or looking at one's watch when another actor is speaking. Organizations, a type of collective actor, also make gestures. The institutional arrangements for psychiatric hospital admission described by Goffman (1961) and by people we interviewed

("They take away your clothes," and "I was given a heavy-duty psychotropic drug and strapped down to a bed for twenty-four hours") are gestures. In the places where people seek access to health and social services, rules (and the sometimes uneven enforcement of these rules) are gestures, as are the uses of physical space (toilets that are off-limits to clients).

In a given dignity encounter, gestures are the responses that follow the actors' interpretation of markers and of other gestures. The social processes of violation that unfold during the encounter are constituted by gestures. When closely examined, each of the social processes of dignity violation I have described consists of one or more of these communicative acts, words, or deeds—the "actions and reactions of others" (Brooker 2008, 120)—that express multiple forms and degrees of disrespect.

Awareness and interpretation are the engine at the center of this cycle of markers, gestures, and responses. All markers and gestures are socially situated. That is, they draw their symbolic power from meanings that are held in common and from being enacted in context. Toothlessness is not a dignity marker in a six-year-old child. Looking at one's watch does not signal disrespect when one is trapped on a stalled subway train. Awareness and interpretation are processes of shared meaning-making and as such can be analyzed like any other social process.

During moments of awareness and interpretation, an actor uses one or more senses to discern a marker or gesture, reads it, attributes meaning to it, and formulates a response to it. Interpretation of markers as indicating a dignity deficiency results in the gestures that express disrespect, demonstrating the conclusion that the bearer of these markers need not be treated with dignity. Interpretation of these responsive gestures of disrespect by the disrespected actor results in the damage that is the consequence of dignity violation.

Dignity markers are material and aesthetic manifestations of dignity status. Markers are assessed through a process of social comparison that includes scanning for markers, scrutinizing the significance of the markers found, and assigning them a relative value. People we interviewed used the phrase "passing judgment" to denote this kind of social comparison, describing the almost instantaneous calculations actors make to assess the dignity status of other actors. One man said:

> It's not like there's a written standard or anything, you know what I mean. It's not like saying, OK, certain people, you know what I mean. If you can prove your income is this much, we'll treat you like this, you know what I mean, and if you can't prove your income we'll treat you like this . . . but yeah, you can look at somebody and say, you know, he's a bum, whatever, let's kick him to the curb.

A woman described how bus drivers react to different kinds of passengers:

> A thirty-five-year-old White woman asks for directions and she's given it very clearly. A forty-two-year-old haggard immigrant not speaking very well asks for directions and the driver just says, "Go over there," and slams the door. And it's clear to me "go over there" means nothing . . . because there's nothing over there.

As these quotations suggest, assessments of markers that produce low estimations of an actor's dignity status result in poor treatment—the gestures that make up violation processes like rudeness, disregard, diminishment, exclusion, and contempt. Judgments passed in the past often carry into the present and future; to be undone, something must prompt the undertaking of a new assessment. Many judgments are also transitive: judgments of groups are applied to individuals, and judgments of individuals are applied to whole groups.

Intersubjectivity—the notion that we become aware of and interpret our selves through the eyes of others (Cooley [1902] 1983; Goffman 1961; G. H. Mead [1934] 1962; Tunstall 1985; Honneth 1995)—is helpful to understanding the mechanism that links the awareness and interpretation of gestures, and the damage that results from dignity violation. George Herbert Mead argued that while we have an immediate knowledge of "the I," or the self as subject, our knowledge of "the me," or the self as object, requires that we come to see ourselves as others do. In a dignity encounter, each actor is simultaneously making and interpreting gestures. Interpreting the gestures of others also involves a process of coming to understand the meaning that one's own gestures have for the other actor (Honneth 1995). Gestures made by self and others are "'read' by self and other for the image of self they imply" (Goffman 1961, 47). Gestures of disrespect are interpreted as "an expression of the state that [the] self has fallen to" (ibid., 149). The actor comes to own the lack of dignity he sees reflected in the mirror of others' gestures toward him.

At times, these processes of awareness and interpretation may take place within a single actor. The "I" and the "me" become the actors in a dignity encounter. (One may even occupy a position of antipathy; the other, vulnerability.) The actor does not need to see himself through the looking glass of others' eyes, because he has internalized a "generalized other" (G. H. Mead [1934] 1962) who reads and interprets the actor's own markers and gestures—the indications the "I" makes to the "me." Thus, we see that people are acutely aware of their own dignity markers and gestures. The attribution of having "given up" dignity arises because the "me" has interpreted the markers and gestures of the "I" and discerned some distance between the actual and the ideal self—a standard has been ignored, a line crossed. A similar phenomenon may be found among collective actors. The "hierarchy of oppression" phenomenon alluded to earlier is a result of groups internalizing the interpretations of the broader society.

Dignity violation is socially and culturally situated because awareness and interpretation are situated processes: they have contexts and histories. The conditions of violation I described earlier in this chapter interact with markers and gestures and support awareness of particular things and certain interpretations. Actors who stand in positions of vulnerability that are particularly acute (such as serious illness) or that have endured over time (such as reduced circumstances) may grow more likely to interpret gestures as dignity violations. An audience of mental health service providers suggested to me that people who are clinically depressed suffer from a pessimism and lack of self-esteem that predisposes them to negative readings of gestures. "After a while," one woman told me, the little things "start to build up. I don't know. I feel like I've gotten the sand kicked at me one too many times and it builds up and usually I think that it comes out worse." (Alternatively, people in these positions are sometimes surprised at how their dignity endures, even as their circumstances grow more dire.) The harsh circumstances in some settings structure interpretation. A man explained that on a psychiatric ward, staff members are attuned to particular kinds of patient markers and gestures, interpreting them as symptoms. Because their responses reflect this understanding, and because of the asymmetries of power and authority that exist between staff and patients, the responsive gestures made by staff often result in further dignity violation and more profoundly damaged dignity for patients.

In a social order of inequality, individual and collective actors interpret gestures from radically different standpoints. Different actors may interpret the same set of gestures in very different ways. Some of the high-status professionals I spoke to insisted that people in "one down" positions could be too sensitive—often "misinterpreting" neutral or even benevolent gestures as dignity violations—and that the proper systemic response should be education or therapy directed at helping them not to "take it personally." Members of marginalized groups sometimes echoed the latter part of this opinion, chastising themselves for responding to insults and injuries in ways that made their own lives more difficult and resolving to find less destructive forms of response. Never, however, did they question that a dignity violation had taken place. Addressing this kind of standpoint-based discrepancy, Avishai Margalit (1996) argued that it is the perception of those whose dignity has been violated that should determine whether or not a violation has occurred: "There must be a presumption in a decent society in favor of the interpretation given by vulnerable minorities as to the humiliating nature of the gestures directed at them" (183). Someone who perceives that his dignity has been violated cannot be told he is wrong. It is, after all, his own dignity.

What of the opposite situation—when individuals or groups are so beaten down by conditions of vulnerability, antipathy, asymmetry, harsh circumstances, and inequality that they do not identify violations of their dignity as violations? Pritchard (1972) wrote, "The lower one's regard is for his own dignity, the less perceptive he will be of injustices done to him" (301). Must an actor perceive that he has been wronged for the wrong to exist? Here, witnesses are important. Although observers may not play an active role in a given dignity encounter, they can become aware of and interpret the gestures of the participating actors and decide for themselves if a violation has taken place. At times, it is only the awareness and interpretations of individual and collective witnesses—including after-the-fact observers of historical events—that allow dignity violations to be recognized and acknowledged.

As I have emphasized, the microprocesses of the dignity encounter are, always, embedded in macro-level structures that themselves are implicated in dignity. We can see these structures most plainly in large-scale phenomena like status-based partiality by governments, group punishment, apartheid, slavery, and politicized acts of rape (McDougal, Lasswell, and Chen 1980; Paust 1984) that are enacted by collective entities against collective entities. Such ordered and methodical practices provide examples of several intertwined systems of dignity violation—systems of hierarchy, systems of dispossession, and systems of oppression.

Systems of hierarchy are societal structures in which individuals and groups are sorted and graded—top to bottom—by ascribed and achieved attributes like race, ethnicity, sex, gender, or wealth. Robert Fuller's explorations of such structures of invidious distinction, which he calls "rank," focus on the violations of dignity that characterize and sustain these structures (2003, 2006). "Rankism" occurs when differences in rank "are used as an excuse to abuse, humiliate, exploit, and subjugate" (Fuller 2003, 4). "Rank-based abuses" include such processes of dignity violation as rudeness, disregard, condescension, contempt, and discrimination, which occur in a wide variety of social institutions, including families, schools, workplaces, and international relations. The effect of these abuses is to create "somebodies and nobodies" who occupy the extremes of the hierarchy. For the vulnerable nobodies at the bottom of the hierarchy, the consequences are grave. For the somebodies at the top, however, this system of dignity violation serves their interests by functioning to maintain their power and authority. It is thus perpetuated by laws and rules and, more surprisingly, by a social consensus endorsed by both somebodies and nobodies.

Class is a particular example of a system of hierarchy. The classic sociological examination of class in the United States, Richard Sennett and Jonathan Cobb's *The Hidden Injuries of Class* (1972), emphasized the ways in which class distinction are grounded in manipulations of dignity: "Class is a system for limiting freedom: it limits the freedom of the powerful in dealing with other people, because the strong are constricted within the circle of action that maintains their power; class constricts the weak more obviously in that they must obey commands. What happens to the dignity men see in themselves and in each other, when their freedom is checked by class?" (28).

> Class society takes away from all people within it the feeling of secure dignity in the eyes of others and of themselves. It does so in two ways: first, by the images it projects of why people belong to high or low classes—class presented as the ultimate outcome of personal ability; second, by the definition society makes of the actions to be taken by people of any class to validate their dignity—legitimizations of self which do not, cannot work and so reinforce the original anxiety. (170–71)

In a class-based society, dignity is associated with asymmetrical qualities of independence and ability that are understood to inhere in individuals. Those who have dignity must have earned it, while those who lack these qualities must have fallen short—and thus may be viewed with antipathy. Indignity is perceived as an individual failure to be remedied not by societal change (addressing the structural factors that promote or undermine independence and ability) but by individual action directed at "validat[ing] the self" (75), such as engaging in competition or behaving in ways that denigrate the dignity of others. In this "contest for dignity" (147), however, these ostensible "tools of freedom become sources of indignity" (30). That is, they become dignity traps.

Sennett and Cobb's analysis suggests that those who suffer the indignities of class may still support the system because they feel "existentially responsible" (95) for their own lack of dignity. In seeing indignity as a "problem of self . . . that transcend[s] power" (89), they believe that they can overcome it through individual effort. In this way, indignity becomes a way to perpetuate the existence of the class system: "Society injures human dignity in order to weaken people's abilities to fight against the limits class imposes on their freedom" (153).

Caste, a system of hierarchy found most often in India and other parts of South Asia, provides another example. Although Sennett and

Cobb might disagree, Gopal Guru (2005) argued that caste differs from class:

> If there is only class difference in society, that is, if there is no discrimination on the basis of caste, religion, gender and race, then it is possible that a poor man could transcend his class by dint of hard work, talent and education, and the dignity which accrues to the higher class would be his by rights. . . . But in a society which discriminates on the basis of caste, religion, gender and race, the worth of an individual does not rest on his being part of humanity, but is considered high or low according to his caste. (36)

Caste "is sanctioned by religion, supported by tradition and maintained by self-interest" (Das 2005, 144).

Despite recent efforts at reform, members of the lowest caste, called Dalits in India, find that their dignity is still severely constrained. "Even an uneducated and poor Brahmin [a member of the highest caste] is far more secure compared to a rich educated Dalit as far as his right to 'dignity' is concerned. There is no scope even for a minimal self-respect for the Dalits" (Guru 2005, 36). The indignity of the Dalits—the lack of human value ascribed to them—is symbolized by an individual and collective body that is considered polluted and "untouchable" by members of higher castes. It is perpetuated by assaultive violations to the body, such as rape, which, when committed by a higher-caste man against a lower-caste woman, "show[s] that she has no respect either as an individual or a community" (Guru 2005, 43).

For members of higher castes, dignity "masquerades . . . as honour, signifying political and patriarchal power" (Draft Concept Note on Dignity 2005, 201). The caste system thus depends on inherently comparative and asymmetrical, yet mutually reinforcing, distinctions of dignity: "The definition of the 'dignity' of a Brahmin is partial, without constructing the polluting Dalit" (ibid., 204). Because members of both high and low castes are implicated in the maintenance of the caste system, all suffer a loss of dignity from it (Ali 2005, 78).

Systems of dispossession are societal structures that promote and maintain inequitable distributions of the resources needed for a "decent

existence" (Margalit 1996, 20). Dispossession wields the social processes of indifference, diminishment, contempt, dependence, vilification, exploitation, exclusion, deprivation, and abjection. Together, these
processes violate the collective dignity of groups and communities. Dispossessed peoples not only suffer the material consequences of lacking
access to the conditions of decent existence, they are also humiliated by
the symbolism of their dispossession.

One historical example is colonialism, a system of dispossession that
used the usurpation of land to deny indigenous people not only needed
resources, but also their inheritances of family and culture (Fanon
1963). Another is the "endless circle of disadvantage" experienced by the
Aboriginal peoples of North America, for whom historical and contemporary government policies of dispossession have led to a "cycle of poverty, violence, educational failure and ill health" (Adelson 2005, 558).
The modern welfare state, although intended to act as a corrective to
dispossession by alleviating absolute deprivation, often functions so as
to promote dispossession by reinforcing relative deprivation. Through
practices of surveillance and supervision, welfare recipients are often in-
fantilized—turned into "spectators to their own needs, mere consum-
ers of the care provided to them" (Sennett 2003, 12), a dispossession
of autonomy and status that can be as destructive to dignity as material want (Margalit 1996; L. M. Mead 1997; Arnason 1998; Chan and
Bowpitt 2005). As the Clash once sang, your right to income support
is conditional on your tolerance for "humiliation, investigation, and . . .
rehabilitation."

Paul Farmer (2005) pointed out that the violations of dignity that
result from extreme poverty and other forms of material deprivation
"are not random in distribution or effect. . . . [They] are, rather, symptoms of deeper pathologies of power" (7): "Such suffering is 'structured'
by historically given (and often economically driven) processes and
forces that conspire—whether through routine, ritual, or, as is more
commonly the case, the hard surfaces of life—to constrain agency"
(40). Advocates for the dispossessed argue that the most encompassing
modern system of dispossession—one of the most severe pathologies of
power—is globalization. With its widespread imposition of neoliberal
discourses and policies of free market ideology and economic restruc-

turing, it allows the powerful few to continue benefiting from the constrained agency of the many (Sharma and Bharti 2005).

Just as the Dalit and the Brahmin (and other dualities of nobodies
and somebodies) reinforce their shared systems of hierarchy, dispossession is reinforced by its twin, "destructive replacement" (Sennett and
Cobb 1972), or overconsumption, "a morbid yearning for yet more"
(Seabrook 2005, 147) demonstrated by the privileged peoples of the
world. This morbid yearning—and its symptoms of depression and
anxiety, obesity, and financial and moral bankruptcy—represents another system of dignity violation, another pathology of power: "Neither
a people wasted by satiation or extravagance, nor people denied and diminished by want, can achieve dignity. This is why the concept of dignity pushes forward the boundaries of defining what a decent human
life is. It questions . . . the economic and social structures which distribute their global rewards with such promiscuous and inhuman unfairness" (Seabrook 2005, 151).

Systems of oppression are societal institutions that deploy psychological cruelty and brute physical force to amass and maintain overwhelming power. Unfortunately, there are a plethora of examples one
might choose to illustrate such systems. In this section, I look more
closely at two: the "harsh interrogation" of detainees in the Bush administration's "war on terror" and the treatment of prisoners in the
Nazi death camps as portrayed in the books of Auschwitz survivor
Primo Levi.

In September 2006, five years into the war, President George W.
Bush was asked to comment on the charge that through its treatment of
prisoners the United States had violated the terms of the Geneva Conventions, the international treaties and protocols that govern the conduct of war. Specifically, he was asked whether the United States had
violated the conventions' prohibition against "outrages upon personal
dignity, in particular humiliating and degrading treatment" (Common
Article 3, quoted in International Committee of the Red Cross 2007,
25). "What does that mean, 'outrages upon personal dignity'?" he responded. "It's like—it's very vague" (quoted in Danner 2009).

It was "vague" because the Bush administration had constructed a
fiction to make it so. In 2002, under advice from his attorney general,

Bush had issued a memo declaring that detainees captured in the war in Afghanistan were not soldiers, whose treatment would be prescribed by the Geneva Conventions, but "enemy combatants" who were not subject to its terms (United States Senate Committee on Armed Services 2008; Hooks and Mosher 2005). This designation became part of an elaborate legal justification designed to support techniques and procedures of "enhanced interrogation" to be applied to the detainees (United States Senate Committee on Armed Services 2008). The now infamous "torture memos" issued by the Justice Department in 2002 parsed the conventions' definition of torture, and the domestic law, to determine that these techniques and procedures did not meet the tests of severity or intent that would qualify them as torture; that even if they were torture, such action could be justified in times of extreme threat; and, in any case, that any constraint on the president's choices in the conduct of war was unconstitutional (United States Department of Justice, Office of Legal Counsel 2002a, 2002b).

The "enhanced interrogation" regime was initiated at the detention facility the United States built at Guantanamo Bay, then spread to facilities in Afghanistan and Iraq (United States Senate Committee on Armed Services 2008). Its specific techniques and procedures were products of the SERE (survival, evasion, resistance, and escape) program, a decades-old Department of Defense initiative designed to train American soldiers to withstand torture. Once the "war on terror" began, the SERE training was reverse engineered, with the intent of devising mechanisms for gathering information from detainees (Mayer 2005; United States Senate Committee on Armed Services 2008). The implementation and execution of the regime involved the CIA and the armed forces, including the active participation of military psychologists and physicians (International Committee of the Red Cross 2007; United States Senate Committee on Armed Services 2008); it appears to have been somewhat resisted by the FBI (United States Department of Justice, Office of the Inspector General 2008).

A report issued by the International Committee of the Red Cross (2007) used the experience of one group of detainees to delineate just what "enhanced interrogation" really entailed. The Red Cross report described "a harsh regime employing a combination of physical and psychological ill-treatment with the aim of obtaining compliance and extracting information" (4). Among the "methods of ill-treatment" (8) used were prolonged sleep deprivation, withholding of appropriate hygiene facilities and items, restricted provision of solid food, prolonged exposure to noise and bright light, prolonged exposure to cold, confinement in a box, stress standing (being forced to stand with arms shackled and extended overhead for long periods of time), threats of further ill treatment to the prisoners or their families (including threats of rape, sodomy, and infection with HIV), beating and kicking, suffocation by water (waterboarding), forced shaving, prolonged nudity, and restricted access to the Koran. Interrogation thus was "enhanced" through the dignity violation processes of diminishment, intrusion, restriction, trickery, deprivation, bullying, and assault.

Often, these processes were carried out in ways designed to "increase the humiliation aspect" (11) through abjection. Male prisoners were stripped naked in the presence of female interrogators. While shackled for long periods of time, prisoners had to urinate and defecate on themselves. During transfers from one location to another, prisoners were put in diapers. An FBI agent who witnessed the interrogation of one "high value" detainee by military personnel also reported the use of a number of actions clearly designed to demean and degrade the prisoner: "Attaching a leash to him and making him perform dog tricks, . . . accusing him of homosexuality, placing women's underwear on his head and over his clothing, and instructing him to pray to an idol shrine" (United States Department of Justice, Office of the Inspector General 2008, x–xi).

Primo Levi's accounts of life in the Auschwitz death camp revealed the Nazis' use of techniques that were very similar in both method and intent. Individuals and groups detained and deported by the Nazis to their Lagers (camps) were subject to an ever-increasing series of humiliations and degradations, beginning with the physical deprivations and abjections of the transport (including being starved and being forced to defecate in public), to a camp "entry ritual" designed to [shatter] "the adversaries' capacity to resist": "It is from this viewpoint that the entire sinister ritual [which accompanied the arrival] must be interpreted. . . . Kicks and punches right away, often in the face; an orgy of orders screamed with true or simulated rage; complete nakedness after being stripped; the shaving off of all one's hair; the outfitting in rags . . . it was all staged, as was quite obvious" (1989, 39). Next was the tattooing of a number on the arm: "The operation was not very painful and lasted no more than a minute, but it was traumatic. Its symbolic meaning was clear to everyone: this is an indelible mark, you will never leave here; this is the mark with which slaves are branded and cattle sent to the slaughter, and that is what you have become" (119). The ill treatment of the detainees continued with the cumulative dignity violations of daily life in the Lager—some petty, such as the Nazis' refusal to provide their prisoners with spoons, although the camp had a warehouse full of them, and some profound, such as the demanding, repetitive, and meaningless work that destroyed both the body and the spirit, as well as the many ways in which the prisoners were objectified—their bodies exploited for medical experimentation, their hair sold for mattress stuffing, the ashes of their corpses used for landfill, and the creation of a hierarchy of prisoners, culminating in the commission of unspeakable acts against prisoners by other prisoners: "It must be the Jews who put the Jews into the ovens; it must be shown that the Jews, the subrace, the submen, bow to any and all humiliation, even to destroying themselves" (52). The effect was to diminish, to create a population of "hollow" men: "Imagine now a man who is deprived of everyone he loves, and at the same time of his house, his habits, his clothes, in short, of everything he possesses. He will be a hollow man, reduced to suffering and needs, forgetful of dignity and restraint, for he who loses all often easily loses himself. He will be a man whose life or death can be lightly decided with no sense of human affinity" (1959, 18–19). Indeed, this was the ultimate purpose of the Lagers—a "great machine to reduce us to beasts" (31): "Before dying the victim must be degraded, so that the murderer will be less burdened by guilt. This is an explanation not devoid of logic but it shouts to heaven: it is the sole usefulness of useless violence" (1989, 126).

Thus we see in both the Bush administration's torture regime and in the Nazi Lagers the "staged" use of dignity violation. These systems of oppression begin with an ideology that dehumanizes its victims (Hooks and Mosher 2005; O'Mathuna 2006) and are perpetuated through the creation of the contextual conditions of violation and through the enactment of humiliation (Luban 2009) and of "useless violence," the violation processes that serve to reinforce, and intensify, that dehumanization. Their object is domination (of information, of population) for the purpose of achieving and sustaining unfettered power. They deny the dignity of those who are dominated, yet by doing so, they also deny the dignity of those who dominate. "Which party emerges from the event with greater dignity," Jeremy Seabrook (2005) asked, after the photographic revelations of torture at the United States military's detention facility at Abu Ghraib, "the abusers or the abused?" (147).

Systems of hierarchy, dispossession, and oppression are intertwined and mutually reinforcing. Each system deploys dignity violation strategically. Through the creation of the conditions of vulnerability, antipathy, asymmetry, harsh circumstances, and inequality and the enactment of the entire range of social processes of violation, they facilitate social and political control of individuals, groups, and entire societies, thus ensuring a distribution of power and resources that continues to advantage those who already have power and resources. One woman I interviewed, an activist and self-described "retired First Nations politician," spoke to me about her own growing understanding of this phenomenon: "One of the first things they go after is to remove a person's dignity. And, and I thought, *Well, of course.* Because that's what makes the person feel human. That's how, you know, [they] really start to strip the person. And that's well known. . . . It keeps terrible systems running and operative."

CHAPTER 3

AN EPIDEMIOLOGY OF DAMAGE

A taxonomy and an epidemiology of violations of dignity may uncover an enormous field of previously suspected, yet thus far unnamed and therefore undocumented damage to physical, mental, and social well-being.
　　—Jonathan Mann et al. (1999)

The vocabulary of dignity violation is metaphorical, yet visceral. People we interviewed talked about dignity being "chipped away," "eroded," "punctured," "stripped," or "robbed." (Hand movements indicating either slow destruction or violent tearing often accompanied these verbs.) They offered phrases that described how it feels to live "without dignity": "like a child," "like you are an inch high," "like an animal," "like a dog," "like a bum," "like a criminal," "like a second-class citizen," "like dirt," "like garbage," "like scum," "like a piece of shit," "like nothing." Their language is replete with denotations of (lesser) size or position and connotations of transgression, breaches of many social and aesthetic boundaries.

The fourth and final moving part of dignity violation is the consequences of violation, the states described by this language. What is harmed when dignity is injured? There are some nine objects of dignity violation, or that which may be damaged when dignity is violated. They are: *the body, the self, autonomy, moral agency, status, citizenship, personhood, a people,* and *humanity.*

The material body becomes an object of dignity violation when social processes threaten the structures and functions that sustain life.
A psychiatric survivor described how the multiple exclusionary deprivations of daily life in the postinstitutionalization boarding homes of
Parkdale, a Toronto neighborhood, were notorious for killing residents:
"They have like sixty-five or seventy people living in that house depend-
ing on how many cots they can get into a room. Hundreds of workers
coming in, people dying like premature deaths, regularly coroners coming and saying natural causes. Well, hello, it's not natural to have pneu-
monia at age twenty-seven and die, right?"

Bullying and assault also wreak havoc on the body. A transgender
woman described her encounter with hospital guards: "They said,
'Don't you fucking come back here again,' and wham, right in the face.
And they coldcocked me. I fell down unconscious two inches from a
parking block. Laceration on my head. They probably could have killed
me if I had hit the parking block. Just fell down like a sack of potatoes,
and they broke my teeth." Years later "I'm still in pain."

The body is an actual and symbolic frontier, delineating the bound-
ary between self and other. This body may be violated by social processes of objectification and intrusion that disturb privacy or modesty:

> This one particular man . . . probably in his fifties at the time,
> but he, because of a severe brain injury when he was young, from
> being beaten up by his father, his behavior is like an eight-year-old
> most of the time. . . . He showed up at one of the [programs] at the
> church and told one of the volunteers there that he had cigarette
> burns on his arms and they asked him where he got them and he
> said he got them at his lodging home. . . . I went over to the lodging
> home and the lodging home operator was absolutely, what's the
> word I'm looking for? Well, she denied everything. . . . She got
> out all these photographs [of the man] and started passing them
> around . . . and there was a picture of him taken in the kitchen
> in his underwear and he was kind of doubled over because he
> was obviously very embarrassed. And I asked, "Why, what's
> this about?" And she said when she got the word that he'd been
> accusing her of burning his arms with cigarettes she just stripped
> him in the kitchen and took a picture of it . . . to prove that he

didn't have burns on his arms. . . . The fact that she would just tell him to take off all of his clothes in the kitchen, and stand there while he had his picture taken, was a bit above the most opposite of dignity that you could have, and with someone with his abilities . . . who could not say no.

"When you have no dignity," one woman told me, "everything's open to anybody."

The body stands as a barrier against the unclean or tainted. When that barrier is breached, as through social processes of abjection, the dignity of the body is violated. The "abject body" (Waskul and van der Riet 2002, 487) threatens to lead to "abject enselfment" (509), a degradation of the self. One woman, describing how bladder and bowel incontinence among the elderly may constitute a violation of dignity, said, "I think it has to do with dependency. I think to some degree dignity is also linked with self-sufficiency . . . so to have other people do something menial for you [i.e., wipe your bottom] that is culturally disgusting, considered to be disgusting, you know, we do secretly and privately. . . . I mean, that's infringing on people's dignity."

A dignified body is whole. It integrates the material and symbolic bodies; it provides a vessel for a whole self. Pain experienced as meaningless suffering represents one threat to bodily integrity (Pullman 2002). Among victims of torture, physical and psychic scarring may cause psychosomatic dysfunction in every biological system of the body (Wenk-Ansohn 2001) as well as a disintegration of the body and the self, manifested through "disorders in bodily experience," "loss of bodily perception," "feelings of fragmentation in bodily experience," and "body image disorder" (Karcher 2001, 73). Indignity is carried in the body. One woman said to me: "The first thing I feel is a tightening in my chest. A physical tightening and it's almost like somebody has shoved a big ball down my throat and it's sitting there. I don't like the feeling because it's heavy. . . . It's just like being full, but not on steak and potatoes, but full of something that's like cancer and I don't want that cancer to eat at me, you know. I don't want it to distort me."

Dignity violation damages the self directly as well. Many people we spoke to located dignity in the notions of self-respect and self-esteem. In the literature (as in the accounts of people we interviewed), these concepts are often conflated, but may be defined, respectively, as "valuing oneself *properly*" (or according to a set of objective standards) (Statman 2000, 527) and as a subjective appreciation of "ourselves and our inherent worth . . . a positive attitude toward our own qualities" (Smelser 1989, 6). One woman expressed these ideas as a single experience of "feeling good [about you] within you." When this feeling is lost, she explained, life "goes to shit": "Sorry for putting it that way. [But] if you don't have dignity why live? Because dignity is self-respect. So you've got to have something. If you don't have that what have you got? You've got nothing. If you don't have love, what have you got? You've got nothing. You know, you have to love yourself first."

Self-respect was damaged in encounters where social processes like indifference, dismissal, disregard, and suspicion left individuals feeling so disrespected by others that they came to believe that the treatment was deserved, and thus ended up losing the capacity to respect—or to love—themselves. The experiences of being out of work and seeking employment were cited repeatedly as particularly likely to damage self-respect. (As I mentioned in the Introduction, one woman I interviewed told me that even the open-ended question about occupation on the study's demographic form caused a twinge to her dignity because it reawakened her feelings of inadequacy about being out of work for the first time in her adult life. Eventually, after considering the form for a moment, rather than writing down "unemployed," she decided to indicate that her occupation was "volunteer.")

Injuries to self-esteem appeared to be even more profound. People often referred to histories of abuse in childhood—often constituted by various forms of trickery, bullying, and assault—to explain an enduring lack of self-esteem:

> Some people suffer with different internal conflicts. Like for myself . . . I grew up in a very abusive world. I had no touch of love or sensitive feeling from any other adult around my life . . . and so I grew up with a total loss of self-esteem. I spent twenty-two years in this country and I've gone through a lot because I come with no self-esteem, none whatsoever, and I was under the impression because of how I grew up that I wasn't worthy of anything good. . . . I kept thinking that I don't deserve, I don't deserve, because you keep

hearing it all your childhood, and your childhood paves your future life.

Identity may be understood as "the information that describes who you are" (Reutter et al. 2009, 297) to yourself and to others. This broad notion of identity encompasses several different kinds of identities, including social identity, personal identity, and self-concept (Snow and Anderson 1987). The men and women we interviewed talked about the ways in which violation processes like indifference, disregard, contempt, grouping, labeling, deprivation, and exclusion damaged both their social and their personal identities, thus distorting their own conceptions of who they were. The man whose experience of reduced circumstances I described in Chapter 1 was struggling with the ruin of his valued identity as a skilled worker and an independent person. The financial, physical, and mental limitations of his present "different [form] of life" had left him "stuck," still searching for a self-concept that would allow him to be a person with dignity. For a woman who had been unjustly accused by a neighbor—a dispute leading to both her incarceration and psychiatric institutionalization—the experience of being "categorized and [treated as a person] in that category" by the police and others had led her to declare as dead and gone the person she had been before: "It's sad. She's gone. She don't exist. It's sad. I wish she wasn't. I tried to find her but she's gone, end of her life. They've totally stripped, stripped me of all that."

People dealing with mental health problems or addictions often described a narrowing of social and personal identity that had come about because of these labels. One woman bemoaned the manner in which psychiatric patients often introduced themselves by diagnosis, rather than by name. A man decried the limitations of identity imposed on addicts: "There are so many different facets to a person's personality. You can't just say, 'Well, he's a crack addict' and leave it at that." A provider of mental health services noted that the stigma of mental illness often caused lasting damage to identity: "That feeling that you're looked at differently and treated differently by people and misunderstood, negatively, you know, diminishes people. It does diminish people's dignity and self-respect. It definitely alters their self-concept and their ability to see themselves as equal to others."

In extreme cases, dignity violation led to a loss of any sense of self. One man described this loss as being unable to "find the internal part of you." Long-term residents of psychiatric facilities, the denizens of "back wards," were described by an advocate as "stripped . . . no ambition, no memories, even of a life before." For people who had been homeless and living on the streets for long periods of time, a social worker told me, sense of self was threatened when there was no longer any feeling of "being a part of": "If you lose that, if you are constantly in that place there, loss is a constant thing for you. In the end, you lose a sense of who you are because there isn't anything that defines you in terms of whatever society or whatever group or whatever city or whatever. So there's, there's nothing there to value, left to value."

Much of the damage to the self caused by dignity violation is best understood through the phenomenon of shame. People spoke often of shame, of being ashamed, and of behavior or decisions as shameful. The social psychology of shame (Goffman 1963; Lynd 1958; Scheff, Retzinger, and Ryan 1989; Wilkinson 2005) locates this emotional response in the individual's perception of a disjunction between actual self and what Zbigniew Szawarski (1986) called the "ideal self": a failure to live up to a community or society's standards and expectations as they have been ingrained in the individual (Silver et al. 1986). Shame "is the outcome not only of exposing oneself to another person but of the exposure to oneself of parts of the self that one has not recognized and whose existence one is reluctant to admit" (Lynd 1958, 31). Shame is thus generated through "the constant monitoring of self from the point of view of others" (Scheff, Retzinger, and Ryan 1989, 179) in encounters between self and others, but also in the interactions that take place within the self (or between the "I" and the "me").

For the men and women we interviewed, dignity violation caused shame by revealing the distance between who they were and who they wanted to be, by "throw[ing] a flooding light on what and who [they] were] and what the world [they] live in is" (Lynd 1958, 49). (Many authors call this violation and shame sequence "humiliation" [Lindner 2006; Statman 2000].) Shame was the antithesis of self-respect and self-esteem. It overwhelmed identity and, at the extreme, when combined with experiences of trauma, threatened to obliterate the self.

In their exploration of dignity in the lives of homeless families, Seltser and Miller (1993) defined dignity in part as "an expression of one's intentionality toward the world" (93). One aspect of this kind of intentionality is autonomy, or "a sphere of choices, a sphere of action over which [people] have some control or direction" (98). But dignity violation processes like dependence and restriction may severely damage autonomy. The youngest person we interviewed, a man in his twenties, pointed to children and teenagers as being particularly prone to losing their autonomy:

> I think kids and young people are often treated with very little dignity because of society. They can't make their own decisions and they can't, you know. We have to control them. . . . I mean, it's not always necessarily coming from a bad place. Sometimes you want to control somebody because you want to make sure that they're safe and you want to protect them. But, I mean, you can't protect them from the world forever and, and then you're really not respecting that person. I mean, it's like treating them like a possession.

Similar attributions of a need for protection are made regarding persons who carry diagnoses of mental illness, whose self-determination is often constrained in ways that offend their dignity. I have already described the loss of autonomy inherent in forced commitment or mandatory treatment and in the restrictive conditions of life on psychiatric units and in boarding homes. At the annual Christmas party held by a large psychiatric institution, one woman witnessed patients "being told [by staff members] how much food to put on their plates. Adults. 'Johnny, don't go for the dessert first.' Like who the hell are you to tell someone what they can eat or not eat?" A client enrolled in a program offering a particular psychotherapeutic modality noted how a program provider sought to restrict autonomy under the guise of treatment: "I couldn't take my shoes off in the office without it being a problem. . . . I couldn't take my shoes off because it was pathological. So we had to argue about that and I decided it was, eroded my dignity, my power, choice, and she just pathologized me because I took my goddamn shoes off in the office. So how did I deal with that? I wore slippers."

For adults in western societies, limited autonomy is the opposite of dignity. It reads as a statement about individual powerlessness or a presumed incapacity to choose (Silver et al. 1986). "Dignity is threatened," Seltser and Miller (1993) argue, by a life without intentionality, "when one merely mirrors circumstances rather than acting upon them" (93). As one man told us about his experiences in the highly regulated (and thus low-autonomy) environments of homeless shelters and transitional housing programs, "You just feel like a cork in the water, really."

Moral agency represents a particular kind of autonomy: the ability to discern right and wrong and to think and to act in accordance with one's own beliefs, values, principles, and standards. Szawarski (1986) argued, "A human being's dignity is based on respecting and preserving his or her moral identity" (200). Moral agency is threatened by dignity violation processes like dependence, restriction, trickery, and abjection.

Many people told us about the ways in which their dependence on illicit drugs drove them to do things they believed to be wrong and otherwise would not do. "For some people," one man told me, "it's any way you can": "They'll start panhandling for more money to get, you know. It's whatever they do, right? Break and enter, steal, you know? Others just steal and rip off and cheat and all this stuff and some will do anything." The men and women we interviewed who were active drug users tried to maintain their moral agency by adhering to "standards" or by drawing "lines" they "would not cross." As I noted in Chapter 1, these lines often were demarcated by prostitution (for women, engaging in it; for men, pimping their female acquaintances) or using physical violence to hurt others deliberately. Very often, our conversations suggested that if they had not done so already, people believed they would be driven to cross lines in the future. Yet they seemed to find ways to distance themselves from lines that had been crossed in the past. When he reached the question on the demographic form that asked how he would describe himself, one man said, "I am not a liar, but I have lied. I am not a thief, but I have thieved."

Trickery thwarted moral agency by confusing what people thought they knew, leading to an inability to distinguish right and wrong: "I don't know which is the truth any more. That's dignity. I don't know what is the truth anymore. Stuff that's, that's presented in front of me, I don't believe it. . . . That's how that stuff affects me personally. . . . If someone who sits across from me and blah, blah, blah, lies and bullshit, I'm thinking, just stay away." For individuals confined to psychiatric units, elements of their treatment sometimes had a similar effect: one person told me that being hospitalized "strips you of dignity. Being in a place where every emotion, every action, every behavior, every expression is put into a pathological kind of frame, it really has an impact. It really does. And I think one of the things they do very well . . . is strip people of their own judgments. Of their own ability to judge."

For many, like the man who decried having to lie about feeling better to be discharged from a psychiatric hospital, lying was a form of trickery, understood to be an act that violated the dignity of both the person lied to and the liar: "When you lie to somebody . . . you're not just hurting the other person, you're treating the other person not very respectful, but you're also lying to yourself. Basically, even if a person doesn't find out about the lie, you know you lied."

Survival needs often led people who were "living poor" to religious or faith-based organizations that espoused beliefs they did not share but were obliged to accept in order to get help. In this way, moral agency was threatened by abjection. One man told Andrew:

There's places that I went to once and just would never come back because they just treat you like dirt. It's almost like you go there for a sandwich but you gotta jump through a hoop first. It's like, "OK. Well, we'll, yeah, yeah, we'll give you what you want later, but first you have to, you know, give us what we want." You know, give your life over to God or just sit down and let me tell you about the twelve steps and how you need to stop doing drugs right now.

Another man said:

What's the basic signal? [The] basic message in Christianity is if . . . you don't accept Christ into your life, into your heart, and he was your savior, then you're going to hell. You're a second-class citizen.

The self, autonomy, and moral agency represent objects of dignity violation that individuals see in themselves as viewed through the eyes of a generalized other. They are, in a sense, internal or private. The next two objects of violation are external and public, viewed through the eyes of others. The first object, status, may be defined as social standing, reputation, or role. The second, citizenship, describes a particular kind of status.

Status is damaged when violation processes like rudeness, condescension, diminishment, disregard, and dismissal send a message that an actor has little stature, particularly when compared to others. The dignity-violating quality of a conflict between two students in a vocational training program for disadvantaged women increased markedly when one told the other, "I don't have to lower myself to your class." One woman described how the physical layout of many mental health services agencies, and of one agency in particular, seemed to suggest that clients were of little importance: "There are so many agencies that actually reinforce it. When you walk into an agency and they have staff bathrooms and client bathrooms, that tells me a whole lot. . . . There's an infamous center [in one part of Toronto] where the staff all have their offices on the second floor and all the programming happens in the basement. . . . What does that tell people?"

In scenarios of unjust accusation. much damage is caused by injuries to reputation. The man whose story I recounted at some length at the beginning of Chapter 1 spoke of this kind of injury, describing an incident in which his neighbors witnessed him being taken away in handcuffs: "That alone tore me apart. . . . They took a piece of me, you know?"

For many people who had found themselves in difficult straits, damage to status often resided in the gaps between what they had grown up expecting and the contempt and deprivation that dominated the lives they were actually living:

> Believing as a woman growing up and going to church on Sunday and being a good girl and get married and have kids, and you give your husband, you love your husband, whatever, blah, blah, blah. And I had to hear that constantly. But in the real world when I was out there, it wasn't like that. It wasn't what was put in my brain, because I grew up in a household seeing that. Mother cooked and cleaned and worked and Daddy went to work. Went to church every Sunday. Well, every home is not like that. . . . One day, shit happens. Like, this isn't happening, you know? So what happens, you lose your dignity, because now you're going to have to go to a shelter or

go to a food bank because the money ain't right anymore, and there goes your dignity. . . . There's your embarrassment and shame. . . . Now you're given a shock of reality, which sucks.

Over and over again people spoke of the feelings of "failure" that accompanied their use of services like income support and food banks. In the particular cultural context in which this study was conducted, such failure was often symbolized by the consumption of a specific food product, as suggested by two of the people we interviewed:

When you're used to eating steak and then all of a sudden you're eating Kraft Dinner, there's a big difference, you know?

And the [disability support] adjudicator actually said to him, "Why don't you eat better?" This guy had no money. "Why don't you eat just, you know, more fresh fruits and vegetables and chicken and things like that?" And his answer was great. He said, "I can't even afford Kraft Dinner. I have to have like the, the no-name brand macaroni and cheese, that's it."

"I think the lower you are in life," one man said, "financially, spiritually, mentally, whatever, the lower your dignity is."

Threats to role were also experienced as damaging. Both a young girl and her mother were humiliated when the child was publicly singled out and sent home from school for having lice. Several people spoke of the insults and injuries to dignity occasioned by custody battles, particularly those in which the grounds for limiting parental access were mental illness and poverty. An older single woman was offended when a stranger insisted on addressing her as "Mrs."—"I'm not [a] Mrs., never was and never will be." A man who saw himself as a mentor to others who were living on the streets was offended when a shelter staff member who was much younger than he attempted to lecture him about his life choices.

The notion of citizenship describes the status of individuals and collectives vis-à-vis the state. In his book *The Decent Society*, Avishai Margalit (1996) delineated four types of citizenship—legal, political, social, and symbolic—and wrote of the "injuries to civic honor" (158) inherent in the denial of one or more of these relationships with the state. Indeed, the men and women we interviewed spoke of citizenship as an important object of dignity violation. The phrase "second-class citizen" signified inferior treatment. One man's appeal—"I want to be a real citizen"—was a plea for dignity.

Margalit (1996) emphasized the damage to citizenship caused by systemic inequities in the distribution of state goods and services. This sense of dignity violation was very prevalent among the people we interviewed. They viewed the rights of citizenship, enacted through access to the necessities of life like food, housing, work, and health care, as perhaps the most tangible manifestation of dignity. When access was lacking, so too was dignity. In speaking of being entangled with the bureaucracy of poverty, one woman said, "The more that's taken away from them, the more you lose your rights, the less dignity you have. Bottom line." Thus, the social services "runaround" violates dignity because it denies the rights associated with citizenship. Invidious distinctions between poor and wealthy, as evidenced by attitudes that the poor are "less than [your] neighbor" and by public policies that reinforce these distinctions—such as minimum-wage freezes and very low social assistance payment rates—offend dignity for the same reason.

(It is likely that this dignity of citizenship was of particular importance in the historical era and setting in which this study was conducted. In the mid-1990s, Ontario elected a Conservative government that did much to weaken the province's social safety net, such as the changes to programs of income support I alluded to in Chapter 2. When I moved to Toronto in 2001, and for years afterward, I was struck repeatedly by how the policy changes instituted by that government—and largely maintained, if not expanded, by the Liberal government that followed it—continued to traumatize the populace, and by the ways in which the era came to symbolize a bewildering betrayal of collective values.)

For some of the Canadian-born individuals we spoke with, the multiculturalism of Toronto represented another kind of threat to the dignity of their citizenship. Time and again, people emphasized the nationalities and immigration status of the individuals who had slighted them. This tendency was especially pronounced in stories about encounters with low-level bureaucrats in government social services, in which the injury of inequitable access seemed to be compounded when it was a newcomer to Canada who denied privileges presumed to be inherent in the narrator's national status:

> I don't have anything against immigrants, but this one, this one worker had only been in this country less than two years and was a social worker and was making sixty, sixty-five thousand dollars a year. And I swear to God that this person blew my mind with attitude, right. Then I actually said something that I should never have said: . . . "Fucking government let you fucking guys into this goddamn country, give you a job, give you [a] car, give you [a] house, give you [a] job. . . . You don't know the goddamn language properly. You don't know the English language and you're telling me that you're not giving me any money . . . ? Excuse me. I'm a Canadian citizen and I think I'm entitled, and if you want to argue the point, go back to your own country."

Among the immigrants we interviewed, Canadian citizenship represented a kind of dignity that was often elusive in their interactions with public authorities. Too often, these encounters unfolded in ways that reminded them that they did not enjoy the status (and protections) of citizenship. One man described what happened when he and two companions were arrested:

> Two undercover police officers . . . wanted to see ID. This is in 2002, so 9/11 just happened a couple years ago. . . . Myself, I had all my [identification cards] but not, all my, I'm not Canadian. . . . I had my student card. . . . I had my [health card], my social [insurance card], and a couple other picture ID. . . . So whatever happened, they let the other two guys go, and hold me. And they take me to the station, saying that I'm illegal alien. I've been arrested about forty times since I'm here in Canada twenty-seven years. . . . So they had my name and all of that in the system. . . . They pick me up on immigration charge saying that I'm illegal alien and they searched me for drugs and, you know, and the cavity searches and all that. I was, I don't think that was very dignified.

The African immigrant whose short period of residence in Canada had been marked by continual involvement with the police and courts was completely disillusioned about even the possibility of having dignity in his adopted country:

When I was in my country, Canada is a country that many people [have] respect for. Like, human rights and everything that is like a good, like ecology and things like that. So I have more respect. The thing that I was really attract to come here in Canada. But now [with the things that had happened to him], when I heard that it's a country that people believe that innocent until guilt is just, is just a joke, is just a joke that I can say. . . . The truth that I found [is] that all the system is a joke. There's no dignity. There's no respect. They don't care about people. . . . I don't see any difference from my country to Canada like the way those, those police treating people is almost the same. I can say even better for my country because if you have maybe a problem the police can just beat you and then let you go. But here, they beat you, they arrest you, and they put your name in the high court, and they still following you and things like that. It's like permanent.

Personhood is damaged when people are made to feel that they are not human: that they are something less than human. Often, individuals spoke of incidents in which they were "not treated like a human being" or that left a sense they were "not even a human being." Several women described how the objectification they had experienced during health care encounters resulted in damage to their personhood:

I went for an ultrasound when I was [ten weeks] pregnant. . . . I've understood that when you're in with the lab technician that generally there's not a lot of back and forth. There's no talking. They can't answer you any questions. And while this tech was doing the ultrasound, she clearly indicated that I'd had a miscarriage by asking me certain questions. And so, like, I'd kind of been respecting that like that I'm not going to ask you any questions, but then, you know, [where's] that same respect back? And so there I was lying on the table bawling while she kind of sat stoically and I thought that to be there, you know, and it was like an internal ultrasound, that I felt I wasn't treated like a person.

When I asked one woman what had been harmed when she was objectified by another kind of medical procedure, she told me, "My sense . . . of being a person who deserves some respect and compassion."

People who had been homeless described how the indifference and contempt that characterize the daily round of seeking food and shelter "takes your human worth away." A man talked about how "your dignity being stripped away is kind of one of the worst feelings you can have," a feeling that surpasses the multiple physical hardships and discomforts of poverty and homelessness: "I've talked to a lot of people who are in really horrible situations, but then there's this one small encounter with somebody that affects them much, much more because it's a really deep, personal thing instead of an environmental thing—you're cold, you're hungry. But . . . it's more like, you know, you're not even a human being anymore."

Injuries to personhood often occasioned the use of language likening human beings to animals. While relating the story of a recent dignity violation, one woman used the phrase "being dogged," which I asked her to explain. It means, she said, "to put [somebody] down to nothing, nothing, nothing":

In some cultures people treat dogs, like in my country . . . dogs sleep outdoors and sometimes you hit them with a stick and sometimes they steal food or whatever. And, and it's a custom. You kick the dog. So if you were poking at the dog [that was] begging, begging and whining and looking for food, and you kick it. So we are in the custom of saying you dog somebody when they do that to a human being.

Similarly, people spoke of actions and interactions, like the social processes of revulsion and exploitation, that made them feel "like garbage," "like scum," "like shit." Such language suggests that dignity violation has the power to overwhelm personhood by transforming the human into the abject: that which is feared as other and despised as filth.

The body, the self, autonomy, moral agency, status, citizenship, and personhood are individual-level objects of dignity violation. Violation also may damage collective-level objects. Specifically, it may harm a people or humanity as a whole.

A people is a group or collective entity joined by some common identification. Such identification may be racial, religious, ethnic, or geographic. It may be based on marginalization or another characteristic of social status. Members of organizations or interest groups based on ideology or activity may identify with other members because of their shared affinity. The social processes of dignity violation may be transitive within and between these entities. Violations visited on individuals may be experienced as injurious to the group, while violations of a people also may be suffered by individuals who identify as part of the people. (Margalit [1996] described the latter form of violation as *mediated rejection*: "The rejection of groups that the person belongs to, groups that determine the way the person shapes her life as a human being" [137].)

The men and women we interviewed told us about the ways in which they had seen the dignity of a people violated through diminishment, disregard, contempt, and vilification. Cathy Crowe believed a local official's general denigration of "the homeless" fueled a rash of violent assaults against people living on streets. Mary O'Hagan, a psychiatric survivor activist, attributed the poor treatment of individuals with mental health or addiction problems to a broader prejudice against "mad people," a refusal to see this group as "fully human." Ashok Bharti, a founder of the World Dignity Forum, described several historical and global examples of damage to the dignity of a people wrought by discrimination and exploitation:

> When the dignity of the whole group of people is violated, then we see the condition that we have seen in the south of Africa, when the whole Black population was made worthless. Similarly, the situation could happen like the Blacks in the United States pre-1963 when you know they were not deemed worthy. The similar situation exists in India like when the Dalits have no value, no consequence. So these are the very, very difficult propositions.

The social processes that violate the dignity of a people do so by making a travesty of the dignity-bearing ideals of equity and justice for all. Such violations of the dignity of a people have wide-ranging consequences, including their impact on both individual and collective health.

There are some violations so terrible that their commission can be said to make all of us less human because they diminish what it means to be human. Among these, the literature suggests, are slavery, torture, genocide, and the structural violence of extreme poverty. It is in this sense in which dignity violation may be said to damage humanity as a whole. According to Ashok Bharti, the central tenet of the World Dignity Forum is that if one of us does not have dignity, none of us do. Denying the dignity of others is also a denial of our own dignity (Malpas 2007). As one man I interviewed told me, "If one person suffers, we all suffer in a way."

Damage to these nine individual and collective objects creates the conditions that further future violations. The experience of being shamed positions people to be vulnerable to violation. (Indeed, the one person I interviewed who insisted that her dignity had never been violated told me it was because she was "shameless"—in fact, incapable of feeling shame.) Violations of a people set up and then fix asymmetry. Antipathy and harsh circumstances flourish when autonomy, moral agency, and status are injured. The mutual and reciprocal damage to personhood and to all humanity wrought by dignity violation guarantees that a social order of inequality endures.

Dignity scholars often have observed that dignity may be best understood in the breach. Our explorations of dignity violation, of indignity, teach us about dignity. I have delineated two basic categories of dignity: human dignity and social dignity. The objects of violation cluster around these categories: personhood and humanity accord with the notion of human dignity, while social dignity may be seen in the body, the self, autonomy, moral agency, status, citizenship, and a people. Close examination of each object of violation helps to provide detail to either human or social dignity. An understanding of the object thus improves our apprehension of its category. Too, these objects can be marshaled as the target of practical efforts aimed at enhancing both human and social dignity.

Damage to the objects of dignity violation begins a "dwindling spiral," resulting in "deprivation of the human spirit" and "poverty of souls." "You lose your dignity and you lose your life," one woman said. The first step in this spiral of loss is the cascade of "strong, sometimes overpowering [emotions] . . . shame, anger/rage, powerlessness, frustration, disgust, a feeling of being 'unclean,' and hopelessness" (Mann 1998, 34) that follow dignity violation. Individuals' psychological and behavioral responses to these emotions seem to follow two main patterns: a pattern of response directed inward, described by the men and women we interviewed as "giving up," and an outwardly directed pattern described as "lashing out."

In the first pattern, dignity violation triggers passivity and apathy. It begins a vicious cycle in which the individual "no longer feels entitled to any status other than to be dependent and subject to others" (Moody 1998, 35). "People without dignity," Seltser and Miller (1993) explained, "are individuals without a future, without a project, without hope" (94). One man described this state as "learned helplessness." People in this condition "don't care." They "don't give a damn." One man told us, "For me, when I lose my dignity, I'd be very carefree, lackadaisical. . . . I have no pride, no esteem, everything is just gone, and to me I can feel it because I show it by . . . my body language, my lackadaisicalness, my procrastination." Dignity violation, a woman explained, "makes you insecure. . . . It makes you down and not look after yourself. Maybe not eat properly, not dress properly, not—you have no dignity, a lot of times you don't dress properly for the weather."

The apathy spreads inward, leading to various forms of "mental pathology" (Fanon 1963), including anxiety, depression, and engagement in "risky" (and ultimately dignity-threatening) behavior like the abuse of drugs and alcohol:

> You maybe even feel like, you know, unworthy or unwanted, yeah. It could put people unwanted. It might almost like maybe you turn into like the bum on the street, you know what I mean? Homeless, a wino maybe or a drug addict that you're pulling more drugs than you want to be . . . or alcoholism, whatever maybe it happens to be. Maybe to deeper into that situation.

The culmination of this pattern is, as Mann suggested, a hopelessness so deep it leads to "giving up on life." One woman spoke of her understanding of what had happened when her own mother gave up on life:

> She ended up committing suicide. And it, it was because her
> dignity had been taken away. . . . I think she got to a point where
> she realized that what she thought was reality really wasn't. It was
> just a, a façade. . . . It was just a total abandonment of hope and I see
> that every time I read the paper. I see that, you know, and it hurts
> me. You know, women setting themselves on fire because their, the
> husbands have beaten them and abused them. . . . I understand what
> they have been through.

In the second pattern, the damage wrought by dignity violation turns outward. "Dignity denied rankles, then embitters" (Fuller 2003, 56). As one woman said when telling me about times when her dignity had been damaged, "Usually I'll sit there and I'll seethe." Violation leads to resentment and hostility. In a psychiatric ward, a mental health practitioner noted, "when [people] feel that they're not being heard or listened to and they're just a number, you know, physically it's a scenario where they start acting out. They become angry." Similarly, a man told me: "The little small things are, like, kinda like, those are the things that create anger that doesn't know where to go. Doesn't know where it comes from. Doesn't know where to go. Unfocused anger."

Such strong emotion can be explosive. The men and women we interviewed described the phenomenon of "snapping," or acting out of precipitous anger, under an accumulation of insults, as illustrated by these two people:

> You know, if I'm having a bad day and there's been a lot of bad
> things happening and people being abusive. Sometimes I can really
> lash out at others and be abusive back.

> I've noticed that, yeah, when they are in a situation, instead of
> shrugging it off or walking away, they lash out. . . . I think it's
> become a natural reaction with them when they feel slighted.

In addition to verbal outbursts, denial of dignity may lead to other forms of antisocial behavior directed outward, such as criminal acts and physical violence (Smelser 1989). One person explained:

> They feel like they're no good, and they're, well, my life is all messed up, may even turn into criminals, you know. Well, I'm going to mess somebody else's life up because [I] have no self-worth, no self-esteem.

A man remembered:

> I had to warn a couple of people, "You know what? You stay away from me." You know, like eventually I will . . . it's like eventually I'm going to snap. I will hurt somebody, you know?

When Andrew asked the man who had had the earlier-described dignity encounter with the methadone clinic receptionist how he felt after the incident, he evidenced this kind of response: "I wanted to jam down, jam my hand down the back of her neck and rip her fucking spine out, you know?"

Federal prisoner Greg Hanson, convicted of murder, described the way in which this pull toward violence is part of a "life cycle of indignity":

> The conclusion I've reached is that even though we are born with dignity, the world we are born into is full of indignity. . . . When dignity is first taken from us, we feel "indignant." Without correction, our base response is to take dignity from others in an attempt to retrieve our own. Logically, this "tit-for-tat" model of conflict resolution is the wrong response. It only creates a firestorm of people robbing dignity from others. Yet it is the model we continue to follow into adulthood—often without a second thought. What it creates is a life cycle of indignity as the pendulum swings between losing and taking dignity. (quoted in Jackson and Stewart 2009, 20)

Dignity violation incites a broader culture of aggression directed downwards, in this way recapitulating and reinforcing existing asymmetries:

> The stresses of hierarchy and the effects of more hierarchical relations, of institutional structures of power and subordination are passed downwards. . . . People subordinated by their social or institutional superiors and threatened with humiliation attempt to regain their sense of control and restore their self-esteem by asserting authority and control over those below them. . . . At the bottom, where people lack other ways of regaining their self-respect, the tendency is to try to regain it by asserting superiority over whatever minorities are most vulnerable. (Wilkinson 1999, 266)

"Giving up" and "lashing out" are not necessarily mutually exclusive. Although the individuals we interviewed seemed to indicate some propensity toward one reaction or the other, there was a strong suggestion that most people could manifest elements of both patterns, although probably not to the extremes of suicide or physical violence against others. Neither pattern was confined to men or to women. The factor that appeared to be most determinative of which pattern would emerge had to do with the characteristics of the dignity violations experienced. Violations that involved the long duration of constant dull insult—processes like indifference, deprivation, and discrimination—and constant exposure to the contextual conditions associated with dignity violation seemed most likely to lead to giving up. People used language like "my stone's being chipped away" or "I don't have any dignity left" to describe this experience of violation. Lashing out, on the other hand, seemed linked to a pattern of repeated frequent sudden and short, but sharp insults—processes like rudeness, trickery, or bullying that attain their power in part through their resonance with past violations, as these two men told us:

> When I see people blowing up and it seems like for nothing, . . . it's because of all those little, those little frustrating things that happened in the last month or so that they had no release for.

You lose a lot of your dignity because . . . you're coming in contact with people that have given me put-downs or been abusive to me or just seem to be pressurizing me, pushing my buttons to see if I'll get angry. That kind of thing.

Dignity may be lost either by giving up or by lashing out. "Living without dignity" describes a state at the intersection of an accumulation of dignity-violating encounters and the endurance of dignity-violating contextual conditions. Here, the breadth and depth of damage has caused dignity and "all that" to go "down the drain," leaving individuals "crouched . . . in the shards of a broken life," unable to value either themselves or others. A service provider told me:

People I see at the drop-in are at the point where they really don't have any dignity left. They're malodorous. They are, you know, their teeth are missing. They, they speak about themselves like "I've got nothing left to lose."

Another person noted:

The shelters and that, they originally were designed for just a three-months' stay to get the person on their feet. . . . Now some of these people are stuck in these places for over two years. . . . And after a while they, they don't care. . . . After a while they don't care. They lose all respect in themselves. And I feel that's when they lose their dignity.

"Living without dignity," said one man, "is like climbing up a ladder without rungs." Echoing M. F. K. Fisher's observation of smudging, a woman I spoke to visualized those who are living without dignity as resembling "Swiss cheese," blurred by the holes and jagged edges of accumulated damage.

When asked to describe people who were living without dignity, the men and women we interviewed often used panhandlers as their exemplars. The act of begging is seen to be deeply shameful, and was understood by most people (although not all) as a last resort engaged only when dignity has been lost. Yet as they reflected on the panhandlers they had encountered, gradations of dignity emerged where at first there were assumed to be none: the panhandler who stands has more dignity than the one who begs while sitting on the sidewalk; the panhandler who asks you for money and takes no for an answer has more dignity than the one who is aggressive and follows you down the street; any panhandler has more dignity than a thief. The recognition that there are degrees of dignity, and that an individual's actions may determine his placement on a dignity scale, opens up the possibility that dignity loss needn't be absolute or permanent. Indeed, as we will see, much of what people do to promote dignity is focused on reclaiming dignity that once has been lost.

This exploration of the consequences of dignity violation has thus far focused on individuals and on the impact of damage to the body, the self, autonomy, moral agency, status, citizenship, and personhood. In the wake of damage to a people or humanity, however, consequences also exist for collective entities. Whole communities and societies may be affected by dignity violation. Robert Fuller (2003) described some consequences of "indignity" for a wide range of social institutions: "Indignity in the family stunts personal growth; in the schools, it sabotages learning; on the job, it taxes productivity. . . . In international relations, indignity threatens peace and undercuts development and global prosperity" (132).

Like individuals, collective entities may give up or lash out. When a community or society gives up, damage turns inward, resulting in dysfunctions that hinder social organization. For example, in his reconceptualization of addictive behaviors, Bruce Alexander (2008) posited what he calls the dislocation theory of addiction. Here, the physical, social, cultural, linguistic, and economic dispossession of a community or society leads to addictions (defined by Alexander as "overwhelming involvement with any pursuit whatsoever that is harmful" [48]) that further undermine the integration and stability of the collective. Among the examples he cited are the high rates of substance abuse among members of North American Aboriginal communities dislocated by European settlers and the worldwide epidemic of conspicuous consumption linked to the "unrelenting pressures towards individualism, competition, and rapid change" (3) brought about by the widespread adoption of neoliberal free-market principles and policies. One woman I interviewed described a similar "traumatization of our culture": "People are scared, living out of fear. . . . [There has been] enormous stress for numbers of decades from infrastructures and systems that have caused us to become very out of balance. Some of them were contrived intentionally to put us out of balance, and some of them, they just sort of by happenstance sort of put us out of balance."

Collective entities also may lash out when their dignity is violated, leading to consequences that are geopolitical in their scope (McDougal, Lasswell, and Chen 1980). Social psychologist Thomas Scheff (1994) argued that the collective shame resulting from collective dignity violation, combined with weak social bonds, provokes "cycles of insult, humiliation, and revenge" (3) that account for conflagrations as narrow as the Attica prison riot and as broad as the twentieth century's two world wars. These ideas recently have been elaborated by Evelin Lindner (2006), a researcher and practitioner whose work in refugee camps and war-torn societies has led her to develop a theory of humiliation—defined as "the enforced lowering of any person or group by a process of subjugation that damages their dignity" (xiv)—as the causative factor in terrorism and genocide. As Pritchard (1972) asserted, when individuals and collectives lack a sense of dignity, they are often blind to the injustices they may commit.

D ignity is embodied (Guru 2005; Street and Kissane 2001). The consequences of dignity violation are written on individual bodies and also on the collective body. Following the World Health Organization's definition of health as "a state of complete physical, mental and social well-being and not merely the absence of disease or infirmity" (1948), such inscriptions may be read in individual and collective expressions of physical or mental disease, social disorder, and failures to flourish. Theories drawn from work in the new public health suggest the mechanisms through which dignity violation may affect collective, or population, health.

Jonathan Mann first noted "the direct and indirect contribution of dignity to health and health status" (1998, 37) and argued that the concept of dignity might usefully be applied to explanatory frameworks that emphasize the sociostructural determinants of health. Dignity violation may be a proxy for being subjected to an array of adverse social determinants. As Paul Farmer (2005) wrote, "The social determinants of health outcomes are also . . . the social determinants of the distribution of assaults on human dignity" (19). Thus, dignity violation and health inequity may originate in the same sources. Loss of dignity also may be a mediator of the relationship between a social determinant and health status, as suggested by Michael Marmot (2004): "Greater inequality in society is likely to mean deprivation of education and other fundamentals that lead to health and autonomy. Without these, the individual cannot function fully in society. He is not put in a position where he can take responsibility for what happens to him. He is . . . deprived of human dignity" (1021). Finally, dignity violation may act directly to effect ill-being or poor health. Violation processes like indifference, deprivation, and assault may cause harm to the structure or functioning of the body and in this way be detrimental to health.

Social epidemiologists have investigated the relationships between collective health status and a number of the processes or contextual conditions that fall under the rubric of dignity violation. In particular, population-level studies of discrimination, hierarchy or asymmetry, economic and social inequality, stigmatization, and human rights violation suggest that dignity plays an important role in the associations between social environment and health. A large body of research on discrimination, particularly racial discrimination, has shown a consistent relationship between experiences of being grouped, vilified, and deprived and poor health, especially poor mental health (Discrimination and Health 2006; Paradies 2006). Animal and human studies of conditions of severe asymmetry suggest that enduring inequality and relative deprivation cause ill health among populations at or near the bottom of a wide range of social and economic hierarchies (Marmot and Wilkinson 2006; Wilkinson 1999, 2005). (The extent to which asymmetry affects the health and well-being of whole populations—including those at the top of the social hierarchy—is less clear and more controversial, the subject of much epistemological and methodological debate [Kondo et al. 2009; Lynch et al. 2004; Saunders 2010; Wilkinson and Pickett 2010]. The moral point—that tolerating severe asymmetry diminishes the dignity of all of us—is not a matter properly argued through such technical dispute, however.) Civil servants who perceive they are being treated unfairly are more likely to suffer from heart disease (De Vogli et al. 2007). Group stigmatization, defined as labeling and contempt leading to shame and social exclusion, also has been shown to be associated with poor health status (Courtwright 2009). Vanessa Johnston's research on asylum seekers in Australia demonstrated that refugees admitted to the country under conditions so highly restrictive that they constituted human rights violations under covenant definitions suffered more mental health problems and a diminished sense of well-being when compared to refugees admitted under more humane conditions (Johnston et al. 2009). In our interview, Johnston told me she believed "dignity was a central part of what was going on": "A lot of the refugees [who were living under the restrictive conditions] were saying they felt completely powerless and like they had no control over their lives, that they were just, that they were being controlled. . . . People felt humiliated and really disrespected. . . . That becomes corrosive, I think, and really eats away at them and at their mental state."

Several families of theory have been proposed to account for these findings. Nancy Krieger (2001) described these as psychosocial explanations, which focus on how social conditions cause biological stress and thus lead to increased vulnerability to ill health; political economy explanations, which argue that a society's structures—its economic and political policies and practices—lead to material conditions that adversely affect health; and multilevel explanations, which integrate and expand the other two theories, examining the interplay between the psychosocial and the structural. Each type of theory suggests mechanisms through which dignity violation effects ill health.

Mann (1998) posited a psychosocial mechanism "in which dignity violations are understood to reduce resistance, or the capacity to respond adaptively to a wide range of environmental stresses" (36). Similar mechanisms have been proposed to explain the associations between racism and health (Mays, Cochran, and Barnes 2007; Nazroo and Williams 2006; Paradies 2006) and between lower socioeconomic status and health (Matthews, Gallo, and Taylor 2010; Shaw, Dorling, and Smith 2006). These explanations are consistent with Wilkinson's descriptions of "the social patterning of psychological life" (2005, 61). In Wilkinson's model, "social dominance systems that are about using power to gain preferential access to scarce resources" (75) create status inequalities, subordination, isolation, and other injuries to dignity that through social comparison are internalized as inferiority, shame, and anxiety, and externalized as reduced social cohesion. Together, these internal and external responses—which describe something like "giving up"—create stress, which, when accumulated over a life span, affects the anatomy and physiology of the body.

The leading theory of how social environment induces ill health via the mechanism of psychosocial stress is that of "allostatic load" (McEwen and Gianaros 2010; Seeman et al. 2010; Seeman et al. 2001), which suggests that social conditions experienced as "stressful"—like the inequality-associated dignity violations of dismissal, contempt, intrusion, restriction, suspicion, exploitation, and bullying—trigger the brain to create hormonal responses that affect every physiological system in the body. When environmental stressors are constant and enduring, these physiological responses become maladaptive, leading to such somatic dysfunctions as chronic inflammation—manifested, for example, as cardiovascular disease, and metabolic disorders, such as diabetes. Allostatic load, or "the cumulative physiological burden enacted on the body through attempts to adapt to life's demands" (Seeman et al. 2001, 4770), has been shown to follow a social gradient such that "lower SES [socioeconomic status, a marker for many of the dignity violations described by Wilkinson] is associated with more rapid aging of all major systems" (Seeman et al. 2010, 223).

Theories of political economy attribute the production of ill health to the persistence of unequal social processes and structures that create unequal material conditions. Because these inequalities reflect systemic social biases and other forms of unfairness, the ill health they cause thus can be categorized as inequitable. The structural determinants of the social determinants of ill health, the "causes of causes," are "a toxic combination of poor social policies and programmes, unfair economic arrangements, and bad politics" (Commission on the Social Determinants of Health 2008, 1). Studies of an array of social determinants of health have pointed to the health-reducing effects of economic and public policy-driven conditions such as substandard living conditions (e.g., unsafe housing or restricted access to healthy food) and reduced opportunity (e.g., limited educational chances leading to lifelong underemployment) (Discrimination and Health 2006; Reutter et al. 2009).

These models also suggest ways in which social conditions may structure the individual choices and risk behaviors that can contribute to ill health. Studies suggest that individuals who report experiencing discrimination based on race are more likely also to report using potentially harmful substances like illicit drugs and alcohol (Borrell et al. 2007; Paradies 2006). Research on individual and collective violence ("lashing out") demonstrates its connection to experiences of perceived disrespect (Lindner 2006; Wilkinson 2005).

Nancy Krieger's ecosocial model synthesizes the psychosocial and the political economy theories, locating "clues to current and changing patterns of health" in "the dynamic social, material, and ecological contexts in which we are born, develop, interact, and endeavor to lead meaningful lives" (2005, 350). Central to the ecosocial model is the concept of embodiment, an integration of "soma, psyche, and society" (351), through a process in which "we literally incorporate, biologically, the material and social world in which we live" (352). Thus, the model makes explicit the complementarity between the psychosocial model's physical manifestation of social conditions and the political economy model's attributions of the causes of these social conditions to economic and political structures.

Mariana Chilton (2006) has used the ecosocial model to explain the adverse population health impact of dignity violation. She conceptualized dignity violation as a manifestation of human rights violation as experienced through social phenomena like violence, gender inequality, low socioeconomic status, and discrimination. Acting via the production of psychological distress and high-risk behavior, these phenomena increase both immunological vulnerability and allostatic load, thus leading to high rates of infectious and chronic disease among the groups that are exposed to these rights violations. Framed this way, Chilton argued, population ill health becomes actionable through the legal commitments of international human rights treaties and covenants.

Health care access and quality are widely considered to be determinants of health and institutions of health care are understood to replicate the social inequalities that are endemic in a given community or society. Attention to health equity is increasingly common in scholarly and policy-relevant examinations of health care systems (Centre for Research on Inner City Health 2009; Gardner 2008; Kilbourne et al. 2006). The notion of dignity has been made explicit in some of these empirical explorations. In large international comparative studies conducted by the World Health Organization and the Commonwealth Fund, dignity has been conceptualized as a component of "health system responsiveness," an element of quality of care (Beach et al. 2005; Blendon et al. 2002; Valentine, Darby, and Bonsel 2008). These studies have found dignity to be a highly valued component of health care (Valentine, Darby, and Bonsel 2008); when it is missing in service users' experience, their satisfaction with services, their adherence to provider recommendations, and the comprehensiveness of the care they receive all suffer (Beach et al. 2005; Blanchard and Lurie 2004). Such findings suggest that dignity might be marshaled as a powerful indicator in the drive to assess and improve health equity in health care systems.

This nascent attention to dignity is at odds with a decade or more of a worldwide trend for health care systems to emphasize the rationalization of care in order to enhance its technical quality and to promote efficient cost containment. Critical examinations of this trend argue it may be antithetical to dignity. The structural contexts in which health care services are planned and delivered have features that may violate patients' dignity and constrain providers' ability to do their jobs in ways that promote dignity. Work in this area has pointed out the limitations of health care providers' training, the dynamics of unequal power inherent in health care settings and provider/patient relationships (as well as in interprofessional relationships), the threats to dignity posed by various technocratic rationalizations of health care, and, especially, the many ways in which scarce resources affect the dignity of both patients and providers (Christakis 2007; Copp 1997; Iezzoni 1999; Jacobson 2009b; Malterud and Thesen 2008; Tarantola 2000; Tattersall 2007). Dignity may be threatened by many of the policies and practices resulting from this structural context, including the implementation of clinical guidelines as a tool for structuring care practices (Christakis 2007), the use of "medical necessity" as a criterion for determining the scope of services provided (Iezzoni 1999), and the increasing influence of for-profit ("bottom-line") thinking in even public health care systems (Tattersall 2007).

Our interviews suggested that dignity is problematic for many users of health care services, but particularly so for those marginalized by their health or social status, who appear to be at highest risk of experiencing dignity violation processes like indifference, dismissal, disregard, contempt, objectification, grouping, and labeling in health care settings. Among the effects of the violations described by the people we interviewed were incorrect diagnoses, unnecessary tests, failures to receive the correct treatment, and wasted time and resources resulting from these errors. As a result, people reported engaging in highly inefficient quests for responsive providers and effective treatment. The ultimate consequence was their poor health.

Discrimination and deprivation can manifest as total denial of care, such as in decisions by providers or facilities not to provide services to addicts or persons with mental health diagnoses. Even less blatant violations can have similar effects. Research conducted by Streethealth, an organization that offers health and social care services to homeless and underhoused populations in Toronto, found that 40 percent of respondents in a citywide survey of homeless people reported that they had been "judged unfairly or treated with disrespect" by a health care provider within the last year (Khandor and Mason 2007, 42). We have seen that such incidents involve the social processes of rudeness, indifference, disregard, objectification, labeling, discrimination, and even assault. (Indeed, Streethealth reported that some 5 percent of respondents had been beaten up or physically attacked by hospital security guards.) Such experiences constitute a major barrier to accessing and using appropriate health care: "Discrimination and poor treatment indicates that, at best, many homeless people are still not having their health problems taken seriously or investigated adequately. At worst, it means that they may not be having their health problems treated at all" (42).

In our interviews, many people indicated that they now avoided certain providers or facilities because they had been treated so badly in the past. In systems and locales where choice is limited, the decision to avoid is often a de facto determination to go without care. The literature confirms that individuals who are experiencing stigmatized symptoms or disorders are less likely to seek proper diagnosis and treatment (Courtwright 2009). Dignity violation in health care thus becomes a driver of continuing health inequity.

Discussions of the mechanisms that link social conditions to population health status engage both symbolic and material explanations

(Kawachi, Adler, and Dow 2010). Psychosocial theories focus on the symbolic value of various forms of status and the health impact of the ways in which individuals interpret and respond to the meaning of their own places in the social hierarchy (McEwen and Gianaros 2010; Seeman et al. 2010). Theories of political economy emphasize the material effects of absolute scarcity and the damage that scarcity wreaks on individual and collective bodies (Farmer 2005). Wilkinson noted that the difference between the two explanations "hinges on whether the health impact is dependent on some conscious or unconscious perception or cognitive processing, or whether, in contrast, it affects health regardless of what we think or feel or know" (2005, 61). He reconciled the two by arguing that psychosocial pathways are always grounded in material factors. (For example, the interpretive symbolism of the psychosocial approach ultimately rests on a neurobiological explanation that is highly materialist.) Ecosocial theory, too, suggests that symbolism and materialism are intertwined (Krieger 2005).

This distinction between symbolic and materialist theories, and their reconciliation, raises, once again, the role of perception in dignity violation and the question of whether a violation must be recognized for damage to occur. Psychosocial theories provide a satisfying explanation for how the microprocesses of dignity violation—awareness and interpretation—can lead from the experience of social processes like disregard and suspicion to damage to the individual and collective objects of dignity violation. Theories of political economy show that such microprocessing is not always necessary, however. The damage wrought by dignity violation also may occur directly, through the material effects of such violation processes as deprivation or assault. Multilevel theories, like the ecosocial model, suggest the ways in which perception is always structured by political and economic conditions. That is, such theories reinforce the argument that all dignity encounters, and their consequences, are embedded in a broader social order.

CHAPTER 4

DIGNITY PROMOTION
The Ordinary Language of Respect

> *Human dignity draws its moral force not from a*
> *particular and well-defined philosophical conception*
> *but from the intuitive appeal of the ordinary language*
> *of respect for the human person and her inherent*
> *worth.*
> —Gerhold K. Becker (2001)

You could be forgiven for feeling bleak right now. There are so many ways to violate dignity, so many systems in place that perpetuate violation. Most of our conversations about dignity, in scholarship and in our daily lives, focus on how dignity may be threatened or lost. Explicit attention to dignity promotion is more of a novelty, but it is important to recognize that dignity does not just claim victims of violation: it also has agents of promotion. We had to draw out the people we interviewed to get them to reflect on dignity promotion. Once so prompted, however, we found many (although not all) of the men and women we spoke with had something to tell us about the ways in which the expressive performance of respect can foster a mutual valuing of self and other and may help to establish the conditions necessary for "a dignified life."

The exploration of dignity promotion I begin in this chapter is meant to restore the constructive power of agency to dignity, to remind us of the varieties of purposeful individual and collective action and interaction that can achieve both human and social dignity. By emphasizing the ways in which dignity may be cultivated, I hope this exploration will begin to suggest a way forward toward a more dignified world.

A woman in her sixties, living in subsidized housing with her grandchildren and receiving income support from the province, told me she had prepared for our interview by looking up the word "dignity" in the dictionary and reflecting on its changing meanings and uses in her own life:

> It sums up honor, choice. . . . I thought about it over the week and I can recall back to when I [was] five or six. . . . I certainly felt the implications of what it was . . . I was brought up in an upper-middle-class family. It was a different era then and it was just after the war and so I can remember my dad's army boots and trying to walk in them and, you know, the fact of being proud, you know, for my country. . . . I remember being told that it was manners which were dignified. . . . Then I got into my teens, it changed. . . . You always have some sort of hardship going through school, you know, you don't fit in the group or, you know, kids making fun of you and I always felt it would be dignified to hold up my head in honor, you know . . . to realize that I was a human being. . . . I always felt proudness in myself. . . . As I got older and I had my children, it was a different story. Dignity was, you know, providing for my family, keeping them clean, you know, having pride within one's self and how you're raising a family. . . . Even the simple things like making a meal, you know, I would try to do it with dignity. This is my role, my honor, to provide for my family and to do that. . . . It's an important word to me. It's raised me. It's been, it's been so much a part of me. It's gotten me through hardships, through depression, through shame, through—I've been put down because of one situation or another and, you know, to hold onto my dignity has really, has kept me going.

"Dignity is, is not a passive process," one man told me. "It has to be earned. It has to be asserted. And it has to be communicated." Another person said, "It doesn't just happen. You don't just give dignity. You don't just get your dignity. You hold onto it. . . . You have to continue to feed it." Just as there are social processes of dignity violation, so too may dignity be promoted by action and interaction.

Dignity is promoted when actors' encounters are characterized by *courtesy*. One woman described the social process of courtesy as a set of "unwritten rules" that when followed demonstrate an attitude of "always being conscious of the next person's feelings." Courtesy is important to dignity in the workaday world of small interactions. A woman noted the differences in experience between dealing with automated phone systems and rude clerks and dealing with the rare customer service personnel who are "pleasant" and "patient." A man who had made his living delivering furniture talked about how he tried to dignify himself and his clients:

> First of all, I'd be polite. I wouldn't overstep my bounds. If I was in their house, I would respect their place. I would always ask permission to enter. I would always ask permission to use the bathroom or, you know, use something that they had or that kind of thing. I'd always ask first and be polite. Always say please and thank you. And especially if they were older than me. I always respect my elders. I was always taught that.

Courtesy also matters in families. A mother sought to impart lessons about dignity to her children by teaching them what she called "the basics": "How you speak to each other. Using manners as a form of dignifying each other. Treat each other well. You have something to say—if you don't have anything nice to say, don't say anything. Better to be silent than to hurt another. We have dogs and cats and treating [them with] value and dignity. . . . Treating your teachers [with] respect. That kind of thing."

In health care settings, dignity is enhanced through small courtesies like polite address or greetings and mannerly (and timely) responses: "For instance, if you're in a hospital bed and you're totally incapable of doing anything for yourself and you ask for a bedpan and it was brought to you and you say thank you and they say you're welcome. . . . Nobody wants to use a bedpan and [giving them] is probably not the best job in the world, but that's their job and they've picked it, so let's handle it nicely." Individual health care providers can be courteous: "That's what I love about my current family doctor. . . . I mean, he respects where I'm from, what my living situation is, what my conditions are. . . . He speaks to me with respect. . . . The way he talks, not talking down to me, but talking directly to me and, you know, if I don't understand something, then taking the time to explain it." The total environment of a health care organization also can be courteous: "You go in there and people are coming in there and like people that come in there they are drug users and people like that. They treat you just like you're a regular member of society. They give you what you need, you know, what you need. They are always polite. . . . All the people in there are polite and they deal with respect and what not and of course dignity, right?"

Recognition incorporates attention and validation. Through recognition, people see and acknowledge the humanity and the individuality of others, that which makes the other valuable. A grandmother seeks to build up the dignity of her granddaughter by trying "to pick out everything that's good, good about her. . . . So every time I see her, I say, 'You're beautiful, but what's even more special is that you're sweet and you're kind.'" Pediatrician Morris Wessell described how he always made a point of complimenting his patients, seeking to notice things like new shoes that made children feel proud. A man's dignity is promoted when a counterman at his regular diner gives him a free cup of coffee, noting that the customer is always helping him by tidying the area where he sits. "For him to notice in the midst of everything," the man says, "tells you that he's paying attention." A patient feels recognized when her concerns are "taken seriously"—heard and acted upon—by her health care providers. A social worker suggests to a group of young people that the most important thing they can do when meeting a homeless person on the street is not to give money, but to "give a hello, because you're probably the only person who will have said hello, will have acknowledged that person, and just saying hello makes that person feel human."

Social processes of recognition can be marshaled to prevent or to limit the damage to dignity threatened in difficult situations. In the midst of a lengthy psychiatric hospitalization, a man felt recognized when another patient complimented him:

[The patient] came up to me and said, "You take wonderful photographs. And I know I'm crazy, but I know you're not crazy. And I don't know why the doctors have you here." OK. That was a moment where, where someone was elevating me up and giving me dignity. . . . You're on a psychiatric unit and you feel like you're just like everybody else. You're probably a week into hospitalization, the heavy-duty antipsychotics, so it's nice to have someone come in and say that.

A young woman who was working for a disabled individual described what happened when her employer became ill and soiled herself at a time when the home care provider, who usually responded to the employer's personal hygiene needs, was absent:

So that was an interesting moment of OK, this is a really undignified situation, right? She has to get naked with me, basically, even though she got that kind of help from other people before. She, it never happened with me and it was just a moment of, like, well, maintaining a kind of casual conversation and just 'cause it was difficult, like what do we say? What do we do? Like, how do I? So it was like talking to her and looking at her and making sure she knew I was still seeing her. I wasn't seeing her as, like, this naked body that I was taking clothes off and on, so it was kind connecting with her as a person in the moment.

The recognition given to groups enhances the dignity of individuals, and vice versa. Shawn Lauzon described how public acknowledgment of his organization's importance had strengthened the dignity of the community of psychiatric survivors, which in turn "propels the organization to show that face" (of pride). A lesbian mother spoke of the feelings of dignity occasioned first when the law in Ontario changed to allow her to marry her partner and then when she went to court to adopt the children she and her partner had had together: "Being able to stand in front of a judge and adopt my own children, it was so, like I was just wearing the big D, right? I was standing, I was dignity. I was dignity in the room, you know? You can adopt your, this child can have two mothers. . . . I was like what? Like am I hearing this? Is this true? Give me the paper, like make sure, you know? I carry my adoption certificates everywhere."

Recognition is often twinned with *acceptance*—nonjudgmental attitudes and behaviors that demonstrate that differences are tolerated, even celebrated. A therapist described her own efforts to promote the dignity of her clients by being accepting of them: "I very much practice with an underlying notion of unconditional acceptance for the client: that I'm not here to judge them. I remind them of that. I really try and strive towards not imposing my own values and judgments on people. Like I see people as human beings who are really trying to and doing the best they can right now with what they have." A man said that he felt such unconditional acceptance when his doctor, rather than calling his reliance on marijuana to alleviate certain symptoms an "addiction" (as other health care providers had done), "calls it medication." A woman who volunteered in a hospice found the true value of acceptance in the challenge of reconciling the bad things people might have done in the past with their need for dignity in the present:

I'll be taken aside by [a family member]. . . . Someone might come [and say] "I haven't seen him for seventeen years. He was this and he was that and he was horrible." And then that person leaves and I have to go back in that room and find a place that says, you know, where I can sit quietly and say, "I've done some horrible things in life. You've done some horrible things. We're just human. . . ." It's one of the hardest things. I don't know if you ever master that.

Being accepted means feeling welcomed and feeling that you belong. A social worker described how her agency sought to safeguard people's dignity by not requiring clients to make appointments, offering them coffee or tea when they came to the office, limiting the intrusions of traditional eligibility determinations and other intake procedures, and building trust over time by "listening" and "learning." In the city's drop-in centers, one man who had been homeless explained, "It doesn't matter what you look like, what you wear, what you smell like, if you didn't eat. . . . It's so much uplifting there, right, for your dignity. Like I was getting information, the food to eat, a shower, laundry free, a meeting place, movies, you know? You feel a little at home, you know what I mean? So that boosts your dignity, you know what I mean? As opposed to feeling strange in a strange place." A woman whose dignity had been damaged through the revulsion provoked by her scabbed and scaly hands imagined a health care encounter in which her dignity would be promoted by acceptance signified by easy physical contact: "It would be homey, you know. And the doctor would come, OK, and the nurse, you know, would either hug you or something and tell you it's going to be OK. . . . I'd go hug you. I'd go to shake your hand and not look at your hands first, you know. . . . They hug me, you know. Doesn't matter what I look like. You don't back off or push back."

Empowerment promotes dignity by reframing people's understandings of the world and of themselves, changing their perspectives and raising their expectations. Service providers told me that they tried to empower their clients by first giving them choices and then abiding by those choices—even when the clients did not make the choices the provider would have preferred:

> Even for [someone who is] psychotic or with schizophrenia, you know, sometimes . . . it does seem like an act of dignity to say, "No. I don't want to take the meds. I don't want to do that. I'm going to do this instead." . . . That was the most important choice for the individual to make and that's the choice that the individual felt best about and, you know, at the end of the day, you know, whether he is receiving treatment, he still is an autonomous individual who has to live with his choices and so, and to have this sense of self intact . . . so keeping an open mind to an individual's choices . . . and respecting that . . . perhaps that is what is in the best interests of the client. As defined by him or her.

Empowerment also teaches, providing people with knowledge and tools, thus enhancing their capacities. It creates opportunities for new capabilities to be fulfilled. A mother whose daughter had been hospitalized several times for a serious illness noted that the practice of giving patients information about complaint procedures, including the names of unit nurse managers, was a good step toward helping patients and their families to feel able to protest should there be problems with the care provided. For one woman, a stay at a battered women's shelter led to an empowering transformation:

> And then I went to [the shelter] and that's when I started to develop more, because I had always thought that everything was my fault and when you think that everything's your fault it's hard to, to maintain your dignity. . . . I'll never forget . . . when I walked in and they said to me, "What was your family life like?" And my family life was very, very dysfunctional, but I was like, "Oh no, that has nothing to do with it. It's just me. Just, like, I have a problem picking the wrong man and accepting abuse." So, yeah, until I started to realize that this was not my fault. I started to get my dignity back.

An advocate for psychiatric survivors called empowerment a process of "creating monsters" and described how economic development could empower the survivor community as a whole, thus empowering individual members of the community to demand change: "Giving people activity, giving people money, raising their self-esteem . . . the rewards I saw [were] people gaining a voice and have some respect for themselves, for their own time . . . so that they were better able to give people grief when they were treated inappropriately."

"Not being under someone else" bestows dignity. In the social process of *independence*, people create situations in which they can be self-sufficient, thus sparing themselves the humiliation threat of having to ask for or accept help. Two things appear to be particularly important to achieving independence: having a home and having a job. Over and over again, particularly from people who had experienced homelessness, like the four individuals quoted below, we heard about the dignity-promoting qualities of home:

> It makes a lot of difference. I mean, I'm just in a little box really, but it's so much better really. It's, it's a home—because it has a kitchen, it has a bathroom, and it has all these things that a home has. It's not a rooming house where you share these things.

> Well, the privacy for one. Not being told when to get up, when to go to bed, when you can go out for a cigarette, when you got to eat,

what you've got to eat, when you can shower or when you can do laundry. Oh, everything.

So with the independent housing you have a sense, it restores the dignity. I can put up my own picture on the wall, you know. I don't have to make the bed if I don't want to, things like that. It sounds small, but they're big.

[If you've got] a key to a door, which is your home, a place to live, that's your own, all that is dignity. . . . I'm not going to tell you anything—you are the queen of your castle. You know what I mean? You can do anything you want.

Similarly, dignity can be found in paid work. An advocate for psychiatric survivors said:

I really see income and employment as going a long way in restoring dignity. That it's something a person does for themselves and they feel that they've done it for themselves, 'cause in fact they have, they've gotten up and gotten there.

Another woman told me:

The only time I'm feeling good is when I'm out there [working]. When I'm out there and I come home and I put the key in the door and I feel that I was productive. Every day you open your eyes, you've got to be productive, and you've got to observe the purpose, even if it's a grain of salt. . . . I've served a purpose. . . . I've got a J-O-B part time, and that's what makes me feel good, and that's what's giving me back my dignity.

Homes and jobs promote dignity not just through their intrinsic qualities—the privacy and self-determination that accompany having a home, the money and sense of purpose that come with having a job—but also because of their symbolism. For an adult in North America, having a home and a job means fitting in. As one woman said, "That's how you get respect in our society, right? Is by being, being like others and being, being independent and doing, like following the norm, right?

And that's what makes you a respectable citizen, is doing what our society is already set up for people to do."

Participation in unpaid labor also may be dignity enhancing. Through *contribution*, people give of themselves to help others or to improve their communities. The men and women we interviewed indicated that their dignity was promoted when they engaged in voluntary activities like attending political protests, picking up litter, and working in food banks. They used phrases like "giving something back" and "making a difference" to characterize these dignity-promoting experiences. As one man said, "Not that you have to do it, you don't have to do it, but it makes you feel good that you're doing it. It gives you a sense of pride, a sense of dignity that you're helping and that you're doing something." (On the demographic forms, people often described themselves as "active." Initially, I was perplexed by this designation, until I realized it was meant as a shorthand for engagement with and concern for others. "Being active" means that the person is making a contribution.) Paid work that involved self-sacrifice for the good of others shared this quality. One man I spoke with described a short stint fighting forest fires in western Canada as a time when "my dignity felt really good, because I felt now I'm doing something for society."

Dignity is promoted by *discipline*. Many of the men and women we interviewed described the importance of "doing chores," such as maintaining good personal grooming and a clean house. Dignity inhered both in the end result—an appearance of being cared for and respectable—but also in the process, the discipline, of taking care. Being reliable was seen to promote dignity. One man said, "When I tell somebody I'm going to do something, I do it." Promptness seemed particularly important to dignity; many of the people we spoke with emphasized the value of being on time for appointments and other commitments. (Indeed, the men I interviewed who were living in homeless shelters often were ten or fifteen minutes early for our meetings.) Several men spoke of having a girlfriend as dignity-enhancing because women "rub off on you . . . good things, you know: don't use drugs, don't use alcohol, clean yourself, eat good." For people involved in street drugs, "staying straight" was a kind of discipline, but using drugs "clean" (e.g., not using dirty needles, disposing of used needles properly) also was viewed as a way to promote dignity, as was teaching others the procedures for clean use. Many of the people we interviewed chafed against the strict behavioral requirements for life in the city's shelter system, but some found value in the regimentation: "Once you get into the shelter and you get the hang of the, of having so much people around you, the dignity start climbing back up again because, you know, you're back into little routine. You eat, you got to sleep, you gotta wake up, and they put you into this pattern, the schedule. They throw you into like a work schedule." One man said, "It's not very difficult for me to feel very dignified in society. Because I conform."

The men and women we interviewed talked about *accomplishment*— "doing the job right" or "going above and beyond"—as a key means of promoting dignity. Some accomplishments are quiet: "If you're able to do the normal thing that society has done and, you know, go to school and grow up, go to work, have a family, whatever. If you can accomplish that, then I think your dignity should be pretty much right up there." Others are showy:

> It's just a great feeling, so I guess I would say that that makes you feel like I have value. I mean afterwards there's other thoughts, but the feeling itself when you're alone. It's exhilarating. The crack of the bat, like when you hit it and you hear the sound and you know it's a home run, or at least it's a triple. . . . God, they're going to be so happy. . . . It does improve in a sense my self-worth, because then I become more, I'm more of an asset to the team because now I'm a hitter.

The dignity of accomplishment derives from the personal satisfaction of setting and reaching a goal, showing that "you have it in you to go after something." It derives from demonstrating the discipline necessary to achieve the goal, and from the recognition that comes from others when that goal is realized.

Past accomplishments can become a resource, a bulwark against the loss of dignity in the present:

> I'm thinking about a client right now who, who recently lost his housing and he's had a number of other struggles in his life around mental health issues and so forth. Things have really been tough

for him lately and, you know, in spite of that, you know, I think what keeps him going is that he sees his past successes, he sees his accomplishments as an individual, twenty years ago and thirty years ago and he understands that he's not a terrible person because he hasn't been able to do A, B, or C and that he does have individual strengths . . . so all of those things make his sense of himself as an individual more intact and I think thereby give him a greater sense of dignity.

Enrichment means dignifying oneself by making choices about consumption or occupation that are self-improving. One woman described how she and her family "consciously look at everything [we] do or choose":

> You got to read the right books, not the wrong books. You got to watch the right movies, not the wrong movies. And I use "right" and "wrong" as stuff that will educate. You can spend a week watching horror films. I'm not sure how that makes you a better human being. Or you can watch, you know, films that inspire you. So, you know, that's another way I go with my family, with my children, with my partner, and we talk about is this worthwhile watching? Is that worthwhile reading? Is that worth going to?

Creating and consuming art is seen as particularly enriching. Making art provides a form of self-expression that leads people to "feel better" about themselves and the circumstances of their lives. A reader described how he used books to "stay cool" while living through the "havoc" of homelessness and transitional housing:

> What I personally do and what I did when I was in the system is . . . I love literature. I love like real literature—I don't mean current-selling things. I have found that was a real incredibly helpful tool because it was something that I knew on my own would help me preserve a certain dignity. Without that, I became afraid I would then be like the other people and get squashed down even more. So literature for me is like about dignity.

Nature provides another source of enrichment. People told us that they took walks or bike rides along Toronto's lakeshore paths or in its ravines to escape the dignity-threatening stresses of the urban environment, exchanging the intrusive chaos, noise, and grime of the city for the calm, silence, and beauty of the verdant outdoors. Like art, nature dignifies by "open[ing] up some space that you didn't have before."

People told us that their dignity increased by "being myself" or "being my own person." *Authenticity* is a process of coming to recognize, accept, and value one's own true self, then of showing that self to the world. It requires freeing oneself from the expectations and judgments of others and no longer being ruled by what other people think. "You have first to be yourself," said one man, "what you believe yourself, and you have to have strong will. You have to be really focused more in yourself than think about other people around you." A middle-aged man talked about feeling dignified when as a young person he gave up the hero worship of "great men" and found his own strengths and talents. Being authentic also means revealing one's real self despite the risks of disapproval or prejudice. For example, coming out as a gay man allowed one person I interviewed to attain the dignity his life had been lacking.

People enhance the dignity of others, and themselves, when they honor and esteem each other. *Love*, encompassing but not limited to romantic love, is a process of actively creating and sharing such honor and esteem, as these two people explained:

> And I remember somebody telling me once, you know, love is a verb. Love is an action. And, really, without reciprocity, without a giving and receiving . . . there is no love. . . . What we do for each other will also have some effect upon the greater good.

> That interaction with other people, those relationships, that's the real riches. . . . The real things are the relationships that we have with each other and with the planet, and so on.

The men and women we interviewed talked about how being in loving relationships helped them to be their best selves. Love made them feel special and valued. It created an identity as one-who-is-loved, is worthy of being loved, and thus gave them something to live up to in their loving of others. For men, in particular, there also appeared to be a kind of social prestige attached to being seen as having "a good relationship with a good wife who loves you": "Because when you go out to a wedding or to a special event and you want your wife to be there with you, and you want a, well, not only just attractive, but you sort of want to be, people sort of looking at you, you know, and smiling . . . and everybody likes you. You're proud, you know."

People for whom religion was important often used the example of Christ and his injunction to "love thy neighbor" as a model for how our treatment of others should be shaped by love. One man, a minister who did outreach work with people who were homeless and mentally ill, spoke of Dorothy Day as an inspiration for the love with which he sought to treat the people he served:

Her challenge is that everybody who walks through the door is Christ and that you treat them accordingly. And it isn't that that person reminds you of Jesus or that person acts like Jesus, but it's as if Christ is walking through the door. So, I mean, that's how I try to live my life and do my work and I fail numerous times every day probably, but that, that's the ideal for me. . . . This is Christ walking through the door.

A hospice volunteer eschewed what she called a "religious connotation," but used the word "honor" to express a similar idea:

Like I think I try and treat people, you know—here I go with words—like [they're] special. . . . It is just something that intrinsically we're all born with, something that makes us important or special, and I like to be able to honor that in the other person. You were born with it. He was born with it, the working man. Doesn't matter what you have done in your life, doesn't matter what I've done, we have to honor that in each other.

She offered an example:

Just last Saturday I was helping move a woman who was in the end stage of cancer, and although she's, you know, morphined up, a lot of pain relief, when we moved her there was pain. From someone who doesn't usually say ouch, she was like, "Ahh!" And I remember stopping and looking at her and saying, "I am so sorry." She said, "Well, it wasn't your fault." No, no. I'm not sorry that I did something to you, you know, just sorry that you had pain. Sorry this has to happen to anybody. What I did was just [stay] silent. I just held her, held her gaze and just honored that moment that she had pain, and for me that was a sense of dignity.

Perseverance promotes dignity because for many people "just surviving" hard times is seen as an achievement. Being able to "make the best of it" or to "pick up the pieces" after a tragedy or severe disappointment reinforces for people that they are strong and resilient, and thus worthy. One man found dignity in his friends' encouragement not to give up: "So it's hard to maintain my dignity, but there's people around me . . . that, you know, when I'm feeling down, they basically say, 'It's OK. You're not really doing anything wrong. You're a good guy so hang in there and just, you know, keep a stiff upper lip and keep, keep trudging away with what you're doing.' That kind of thing, you know?"

For people who are down and out, perseverance means a "willingness to go on and to try and make changes in their lives and, and their belief in, you know, a better tomorrow. A belief that things can improve." A social worker spoke with great admiration of this quality in her homeless clients, noting too that their hopeful persistence helped her to persevere:

One thing that I, that keeps me going in this particular area of business is the fact that I, I meet somebody at nine o'clock in the morning. We work very, very hard to get certain things in place, be it a shelter bed, be it a meal, be it access to finances or access to a doctor or any of that . . . and then at five o'clock I shut my door and I say, "Sorry . . . I've done everything now. I do have to close the door and go home." And the fact that that person comes back tomorrow morning and has faith and has the internal drive to be able to come back and start all over again, not once or twice but over a really long period of time. . . . Most of us don't have the drive to do that every single day. Get up in the morning and know that you're going to go through the same steps and perhaps at the end of day either end up even worse than you were or at the same place.

Dignity may be promoted through *control*. The men and women we interviewed described how they used checks on their emotions and behavior (or, as one man said, "on my ego") to maintain their dignity in situations in which it was threatened or even to salvage their dignity in situations in which it was lost. Control encompasses cool inaction, as well as action undertaken. One man described how he used control strategically in his interactions with disability support bureaucrats, seeking dignity in two ways—to keep intact his persona as a dignified individual and to get the material resources he needed to live with dignity:

> I know some people, you know, maybe they have a [disability support] issue and so they get on the phone and they're yelling and screaming. But that never got me anywhere. . . . There's always a million ways to say the same thing, eh? You know, you can yell or you can be too kind or quiet about it or there's in between, you know? [If] I know I have to call them 'cause I need something or something, I'm kind of asking them for something so I better be nice about it, or if they made a mistake maybe, there's no point in getting mad at them. You might stall them in terms of correcting the mistake if they're mad at me. So you try to be as nice as you can.

A woman promoted her own dignity by remaining composed during medical procedures: "They see me behaving in a controlled way, I think, controlled versus emotional leakage. Perhaps even in a way that will be abnormal. For instance, if I'm going to have something very painful done and I don't scream, you know, then, then to be, to have that reflected back at me and have the person say, 'Well, I know this hurts a great deal. I think it's great that you're not, that you're being so brave.'" As suggested by the previous quotation, dignity resides not just in the effect of behavioral and emotional control, but also in the fact that the individual is able to exercise that control. "There is a kind of dignity in not showing one's humiliation," one person said. A man noted the pride he felt in "keeping [my] composure" and "stopping and taking a deep breath before you react."

A similar social process of dignity promotion is *transcendence*, when people are able to "rise above" the provocations that might cause them to respond in ways that would threaten their own dignity. Transcendence is at work when people refuse to "lower" themselves by matching the bad treatment they receive from others, thus declining to get caught up in an exchange of dignity-eroding gestures. One man spoke of "taking a step back"

> I cannot really control the actions of other people and sometimes you get a bad reaction from other people and people may have heard it and you don't want to feel slighted but that's, you know, and you can't sit there and focus on it.

Similarly, another person reflected the value of ignoring disrespectful behavior:

> Sometimes it's better to, instead of saying anything, it's better just [to] say nothing at all, you know. If anybody says anything rude to me, sometimes I just turn around and walk away.

People may refuse to "own" insults to dignity that come from others or even those that originate in their own actions. A woman told me:

> [My family] still tries to impose on me that I am not as good as them but I don't let that in. I don't let that come in. I just filter that right out, 'cause that's garbage, that's baloney, right? . . . I don't own it. I don't own it. It's their problem.

A man said:

> I've done stuff that I'm not too proud of, which I know it was wrong and stuff like that. I just tell the man upstairs, "Say, listen, I own that, but I don't want to own that." It's that simple. You know, I may

have done that or whatever, but, you know what? I don't want to be, I'm not built for that, you know, really . . . I'm not, that's not me.

Forgiveness is another type of transcendence. A man who had suffered brain damage caused by a physical assault rediscovered his dignity when he was able to forgive his assailant:

> At the time when he came to apologize I was still very angry, very pissed off that he, this guy, took my whole life away financially, emotionally, mentally, spiritually—name it and he did it. . . . When he came to apologize, at that moment for a split second I was lost. The anger all came back, but I think because of who I am, my dignity, I kind of actually sit there open-mindedly [and] listened to what he say, and actually hearing him. . . . If I had no dignity, that guy would have been . . . that kid would have been dead by now and I would have been in jail. So I think dignity play a really good role in my life at that instant . . . because of my respect and my self-worth, my esteem . . . that came together at that moment to actually let me accept his apology, freed that burden that I was trapped in.

Preparation allows people to take advance action to guard their dignity in situations they know from previous experience to be dangerous. Several people whose dignity had been violated in past health care encounters described how they prepared themselves for future encounters, including doing research in advance of an appointment, writing down lists of questions, bringing someone along to help them, and steeling themselves to demonstrate both patience and assertiveness. One woman found that the most effective way to prepare was to limit her expectations:

> My approach has sort of changed in that I've sort of accepted the fact that . . . there may be medical doctors out there, family doctors in Toronto that would suit my needs, but as of now I haven't found one. . . . So that I'll just use him as my once-a-year appointment. I need to go in for some checkups related to my condition and I'll just, I'll just do that. And not expect much from him. And I think that's going to probably help me with dignity and how I feel about myself,

because . . . maybe if I don't expect much of him then I won't be, like I won't be so upset after the appointment.

Preparation may consist of obtaining empowering knowledge and skills. Not wanting "to take any [more] crap," one woman spent years in "self-esteem and assertiveness courses" (retaking the same course several times) until she had "built [her] strength" and was able to stand up for herself in situations that in the past would have left her dignity damaged. Another woman who determined that she needed to leave an abusive relationship spent months preparing: "I just took care of myself. I made sure that I ate and slept properly, and saw the doctor. . . . My mom always told me, if you're with somebody, always make sure you can take care of yourself for six months . . . so that's what I did, to maintain my dignity. I, I kept putting away money so I would never, at the end, so I wouldn't have to ask for any, [so] I could just leave."

When preparation is not enough, many people turn to *avoidance*. That is, they refuse to return to places where their dignity has been threatened or to engage in activities that have led to a loss of dignity in the past or to associate with people who have violated their dignity. A man described using "experimental" trial and error, figuring out how various actions and behaviors might affect his dignity and then steering clear of those that had already proved to have ill effects. For example, he said, "I don't drink because I know when I drink it's trouble" for "a lot of things, including dignity, so I don't do it." Several people told me they did everything possible to avoid interacting with income support bureaucrats, because their past experiences with individuals in these roles had been so terrible. A woman who worked in the sex trade in Toronto explained to Vanessa that she and her colleagues had created a "bad date book" that contained descriptions of clients known to be abusive or violent so these men could be avoided.

For some people, threats to dignity are so pervasive that avoidance turns into total withdrawal. One woman used the image of a bell jar, with a door that opened only from the inside, to tell me about how she had sought to keep the world out in order to preserve her dignity:

It's like a clear glass bell jar around me, but not having a door on the outside and I'm on the inside because for me—I'm not as easily

affected as I once was—but that was a problem for me, where
like some people could just like open the door, dump their shit in
and close it and I'd be like, "Oh, what's all this crap?" and I'd feel
overwhelmed by whatever it was. . . . [But now] I've got the door on
the inside so I can keep the door shut. But, I mean, it's cracked, it
happens, and for me, dignity is an ongoing battle to, to, to not lose
it, to keep it.

The process of *concealment* allows people to "cover up" those markers
that, if perceived, would lead their dignity to be put at risk. People used
the phrase "keeping up appearances" to describe how they used concealment as a kind of dignity protection. A longtime drug user took pains
to conceal her drug use from family and friends: "I don't know if I'm
supposed to say this. This is the dignity: I've been closeted. I've been using drugs since I was fifteen years old. I've been closeted 'cause I raised a
son by myself and everything and I had so much to lose. I just could not
afford that, you know? So that's where my dignity came. I would do the
church thing and hallelujah on Sunday and then call the crack dealer."
Poor people seek to hide their poverty:

> People who are really marginalized have also learned to use some
> tricks to cover up their marginalization. Children go to school
> hungry in this city, and, but you know, nobody knows that the child
> is going to school hungry. Parents find ways to cover up that sort
> of thing by making their children silent about their family affairs.
> . . . "If the teacher asks, did you have breakfast, put up your hand
> and say you had porridge or whatever, you know, sausage and eggs."
> Because the child does not—the parent doesn't want the child to be
> identified as poor, you know.

A young woman made a point of wearing full makeup and dressing styl-
ishly during her lengthy hospitalizations for cancer treatment to stave
off the pity that would damage her dignity:

> It takes a little bit more effort, but I'm not going anywhere so I have
> the time to do that. But I don't, I don't like to look sick. If I don't
> have to. So for me that's just my own peace of mind. I just don't want

to look the part. . . . I don't want to be pitied for any reason. And if I look sick or if something looks off, I tend to get a different reaction from people than if I look well . . . because the first thing I think of when I see somebody sitting in the waiting room, they're kind of humped, you know, slouched over and, and with their head exposed or what not and then I'm just like oh, that person must really be sick and they're not feeling well. And you do, you start to feel sad for that person. And I don't like that. For me personally I don't like that. So I will try and, you know, put on whatever I can to make it seem that I'm doing OK.

At times, concealment may be the last way people have to seem to be conforming to the societal standards and expectations that constitute dignity:

If you think about being homeless in this city, a very basic thing may come to mind: where do you go to take care of your personal needs like just going to the washroom . . . ? There are [homeless] people who relieve themselves on the streets. But you will find that even that, people try and find a little bit of closed space where they can take care of that very basic personal need. In other words, they haven't gone so far as to use public spaces as openly as, as the field by others. There is that perception as well, you know, people who are homeless, you know, relieve themselves everywhere. But we find that people actually try and cover themselves and find, find a corner or, you know, an incline within a building or behind a tree and so they have not lost all of their dignity.

Dignity is promoted by *advocacy,* the practice of standing up for those who are struggling for their rights. Advocacy encompasses witnessing and testimony. Cathy Crowe described the power of being a witness:

You know, when you see atrocity, you, you can't help but feel something and then you have to do something. If you can witness the injustice and, you know, for the purpose of fighting for people's rights or dignity, I think that's what we should be doing.

A man told Vanessa:

> A guard came to court for me and said that I'm an excellent person
> and that I was one of the best inmates he'd ever seen and he stood
> up for me, right? He worked at that jail for like seventeen years so he
> had a lot of weight. And the judge also said that that was first time
> ever a guard has ever come to court for a person.

Advocacy also includes acts of mediation and translation that one
woman, speaking of her experience in advocating for someone in a psychiatric facility, characterized as a kind of bridging: "Sometimes people
need a voice—not to act on their behalf, though sometimes that's necessary—but almost to be a diplomat or an interpreter. I knew this one
person's story a bit . . . and the doctors could not make head or tail of
what she was saying. They were telling her she wasn't presenting properly. They were trying to give her clues, but they couldn't tell her. So
there's the bridge."

A particular kind of advocacy is *presence*, where people are able to
promote the dignity of others just by being there. People often spoke
of the dignity value of being able to "vent"—to unload their troubles to
someone who would just listen. (I believe the dignity-promotion value
of the interviews we conducted lay mostly in the fact that we really listened to what people had to say.) A legal aid lawyer felt a particular ob-
ligation to listen to clients who were in positions of vulnerability, such
as those individuals who were poor or experiencing mental illness:

> You have to treat these [clients] with almost more respect. Like
> our legal aid clients, we have to treat them with, in a way that they
> almost don't expect to be treated because in a lot of cases everybody
> else has screwed them over, so here we listen longer. . . . If they call
> and it takes them a lot longer to explain their story, just let them.
> They need to. If they call and they're complaining about things
> that you can't help them with, just let them get it off their chests.
> That's something they need to do, . . . even if at the end of a long
> conversation you end up saying, "I can't help you with any of this
> stuff." . . . I think it made people feel better to know that at least

they could, they weren't getting a "shut up," you know? They weren't getting, "That's not within my job description so I'm not going to listen to you."

Several men noted that their feelings of being important and valued were enhanced when their social service workers made attempts to stay in touch with them. An administrative worker at an agency that provides health and social services to homeless people noted the importance of opening the office on time every day. She called this a dignity "ritual": "As simple as that sounds, it shows that I, I got in on time because I know you need the service. You're here on time. You're here waiting for me to open because you obviously need the service. I open the door, welcome you right in. Right there, we've got a ritual, a daily opening on time, of dignity."

Presence also may be used to prevent dignity violation. A social worker explained why she often accompanied clients to their appointments at government social services offices: "I may not do anything, but the fact that I'm there makes a very big difference. . . . The [government] worker knows that I'm a [social] worker and I get treated with dignity, some sense of dignity. . . . We're [not] talking about a language barrier . . . we're just talking about a presence. If I am with my client, my client will feel and be treated differently. If I am not, my client will be treated deliberately poorly."

Support, provision of the material necessities of life, helps to ensure dignity. "I think it's pretty hard for someone to conduct themselves with dignity if they don't get the resources [like food, wealth, opportunities, equity] to do it," one man told me. As one woman said, "It's basics [that] give people dignity." Support promotes dignity when it is given with generosity. That is, support must focus on the individual and his or her real needs in a situation—not just the supporter's notions of what the person is lacking or what the supporter wishes to provide. In addition, it must be given without the humiliating conditions or contingencies that characterize the welfare state's infantilizing practices. Support promotes dignity when it is based on regard, when it is offered straightforwardly and with respect. The following small incident illustrates this kind of dignifying support:

I'd split the sole [of my shoe]. . . . It was like flapping like right across. [At the health clinic] I tried to staple it, and [the receptionist] said, "What's wrong?" . . . I explained to her what happened and then while I was trying to figure out what to do with it, she noticed the light go off in the foot doctor's office, so she called him on the phone and then before I was called in to see the doctor I was waiting to see, she says, "Oh, leave your shoe," you know, "Dr. So-and-so is going to fix it because he has contact cement there." And the last thing I would have thought to ask for was the exact thing that— because you're in a doctor's office, you know—so the last thing I expected to find there was like, you know, was contact cement . . . the exact thing you would use to, you know, repair the problem. So the, the foot doctor repaired my shoe while I saw the other doctor, which I thought was like just, you know, oh geez, I felt like, I felt like, I felt like royalty, you know?

Advocacy, presence, and support operate not just in encounters between professional helpers and their clients, but also in the relationships between and among marginalized individuals and groups. A number of the men and women we interviewed who were living in difficult circumstances talked about the ways in which they and others in their social circles enacted these processes for each other. A man told Andrew:

Some people say I'm a walking encyclopedia because I know more about the system of welfare and missing the red tape and my social worker says I could become a social worker because I know what's, what, what is offered to the people . . . and I'll advise, like a lot of times someone says, "I got cut off the system," and I won't just say call [your local member of provincial parliament] or something like that. I'll say, "This is how [to work] through the channels" and this and that, you know, and mention the way I tell them to do it, right . . . ? So I feel doing stuff like that for people [helps] them get back into society.

Another person described how he had helped a fellow shelter resident:

> A lot of times I'll, I'll take people out of this area to go to where I
> know I've been treated good. . . . I actually just took my friend that's
> out of the hospital to [a community health center]. And they fixed
> him up.

Through the acts of advocacy, presence, and support—exemplified by
the informal social work and the sharing of dignity maps (Jacobson,
Oliver, and Koch 2009) described in these quotations—people told us
that they not only promoted the dignity of others, they also enhanced
their own dignity.

Leveling promotes dignity by minimizing asymmetry, or what Mary
O'Hagan decried as "hierarchies of humanness." Such asymmetries
may be blatant structural gulfs of power and prestige. They may also be
subtle: the quiet messages signaling that some individuals and groups
are less valuable or worthy than their fellows. One outreach worker
described using humor, particularly self-deprecating jokes, to level relationships with the people he was seeking to serve. In workplaces, dignity is promoted when employers and employees engage in what one
man described as "a back and forth exchange of ideas" that suggests
equality, rather than communicating with one another through dictate
or argument. Several people told us that their legal aid lawyers provided
services in ways that made them feel like anyone else visiting a lawyer—
"like I was a normal citizen," said one man. When I told her about this,
the lawyer I interviewed explained that as students they are trained to
treat all clients (paying and legal aid-subsidized) the same. She talked
about how being willing to share aspects of her own life helped her to
establish mutuality with her clients:

> I would talk to them if they asked me questions about myself. I
> wouldn't say "that's none of your business" as long as it wasn't super-
> personal. . . . I would talk to them about my family and my life and
> how I felt. . . . And I found that if I talked to them not like a lawyer
> but like a person, that helped a lot, too. . . . So I'd have conversations
> with them, you know. We'd go to court and I would sit with my
> clients and talk to my clients as opposed to talking to the other
> lawyers the whole time. I found I had fun with a lot of my clients.
> We got along really well. We had good relationships.

In health and social care settings, leveling may be accomplished by sharing information (minimizing asymmetries of knowledge) and eschewing invidious distinctions in order to treat everyone with the same respect—most importantly, making sure that access to care is not contingent on dignity markers. Social service agencies can provide support in ways that do not humiliate recipients by marking them as needy. For example, an outreach worker explained that his organization had shifted from giving purpose-made vouchers for a local grocery store to providing gift cards purchased from a larger corporate chain supermarket because "there's no way of knowing [whether] you got it as a gift, bought it for yourself, whatever. . . . It's a little thing, but I think just trying to be respectful in the way that you treat people even though you are helping them behind the scenes. . . . They don't have to experience the shame of [other people] knowing that they got it for free."

Leveling may not require such deliberate acts. One woman told me that one summer when an ice cream truck made frequent visits to the grounds of the psychiatric hospital where she worked, it had the effect of enhancing the dignity of the hospital's patients just because "it's so normal, right?" The patients' enjoyment of a cold treat on a hot day was leveling because it emphasized the ways in which they were just like anyone else.

Finally, dignity may be promoted through *resistance*, when people forcefully seek to oppose threats to their dignity or to redress outright injuries. Resistance means saying "no" or saying "no more." The men and women we interviewed talked about "standing up for themselves" in a variety of situations: refusing to be humiliated by an unpleasant and power-hungry probation officer, refusing to wear hospital garb on a psychiatric ward, refusing to plead guilty to a crime they didn't commit, refusing to give up custody of a child, refusing to stay in an abusive relationship. One woman described how she was able to resist the dignity-denying effects of deprivation: "I deserve to have housing. I deserve to have employment if I want. I deserve to have food. I deserve clothes. I deserve opportunities. You don't have to have a big ego to understand that you deserve those things, you just don't have them. There's no reason that my self, my self-belief or the level of my, that I feel I deserve to have dignity should go down because I don't have those things." Activist Cathy Crowe talked about how residents of Toronto's "Tent City" (a squatters' camp of homeless people that sprang up near the downtown core) had resisted in the days before their community was dismantled:

> When people get angry enough, you know, they fight back and reclaim some of their dignity. There's one example from the period of time when Tent City was in existence when the [local conservative tabloid newspaper] wrote editorials or articles about people down there eating squirrels and eating wild animals and two of the people from there actually wrote back to the [paper] . . . saying, "You know, just because we're homeless doesn't mean we eat animals. In fact, this is what we do: we feed them and we've named the ducks" and things like that.

Many people spoke of the positive effects of resistance. Demanding the respect of others helped them to achieve or regain their self-respect. As with several of the other social processes of dignity promotion, this effect relied on a dual mechanism: dignity was promoted through the material results of the resistance and also through the symbolism of having resisted.

However, in people's stories, resistance often had a darker side, that of "snapping." In this way, resistance presented its own risk: the dignity trap. On psychiatric wards, resistance was often interpreted as a symptom or as "acting out," leading to what one person described as an enduring reputation as "a very bad patient," with all that entailed in terms of future actions and interactions, or to what another called "a Jack Nicholson moment" of restriction or assault.

A dignity encounter is any human interaction that results in a dignity outcome. When examined more closely, the encounters constituted by one or more of the social processes of dignity promotion I have described here reveal the presence of microprocesses that parallel those found in encounters that lead to violation. Dignity promotion also involves perception—the cyclical process of awareness and interpretation of and response to markers and gestures. Some of the markers found in dignity promotion encounters include visible signs

of privilege—neat and clean clothing, good teeth, and an upright posture indicative of pride in self. (Individuals bearing these markers will
be seen as dignified and thus will be treated with dignity.) Dignity-
promoting gestures include making eye contact, engaging in easy and
appropriate physical contact (such as a handshake), smiling, and employing verbal expressions of respect (such as friendly greetings and the
use of preferred appellations of address). Specific markers and gestures,
and the interpretations that determine responses, are embedded in a set
of conditions that parallel those seen in dignity violation encounters:
the positions of the individual or collective actors in the encounters, the
nature of the relationship between the actors, the characteristics of the
setting in which the encounter takes place, and the broader social order
in which all these other conditions are situated.

Dignity promotion is facilitated when one actor is in a *position of
confidence*. That is, when the actor is living with physical and moral integrity and courage, is positive and optimistic, and has the knowledge,
skills, and material resources needed to thrive. People in positions of
confidence see themselves as good and worthy and are able to discern
the goodness and worth in others. The men and women we interviewed
told us over and over again that dignity is mirrored. "You have to behave
with dignity in order to be treated with dignity," said one woman. Another noted "the domino effect" of dignity: "If you treat yourself with
respect, it will be easier for others to treat you that way as well." A man
explained that it is also necessary to have dignity to treat others with
dignity, noting that outreach workers who lack a sense of their own dignity find "[their] own problems and feelings coming out in [their] work."

Several people described the roles that education and wealth play in
placing individuals in positions of confidence:

> When you're educated, you have some—you can improve your
> judgment and you won't be naïve and you can understand many
> things. So, and then you can—if there's a problem, you know how to
> face the problem.

> If you come from a lot of money, you've got more options.

> Where money walks, dignity is trailing behind on a leash.

Previous experiences of being treated with dignity (such as being seen and heard), and thus of being dignified in one's own eyes, are important to helping actors reach the positions of confidence from which they will engage in future social processes of dignity promotion.

Actors in a *position of compassion* are patient, kind, and honest. They demonstrate understanding, an awareness of others' difficult situations, and sensitivity to how those situations may threaten dignity. We heard several examples of powerful people who were able to act from positions of compassion:

[The doctor] sent me right down for, what you call, an ultrasound, and [they found] a deep vein thrombosis the size of a football. It was pretty crazy. Then him and the head of cardiology told me I might have an embolism. I may not make it. . . . They brought me a phone, told me I might want to make some phone calls. And I thought it was so kind of them to be honest and forthright with me. You talk about dignity, you know what I mean? They could have pulled the wool over my eyes . . . but no.

[My doctor] put me on testosterone, because my testosterone level was low, 'cause I'm getting old. And if you're over fifty, they charge you for the prostate exam, which you need before he can put you on that drug. Rather than saying this is going to cost you blah, blah, blah. He said, "I know you can't afford it. Here's thirty dollars, go and get this test done." You know . . . that to me is like just someone, just someone who's showing an understanding of where his patient is in life.

[Some judges] seem to understand these issues pretty well. They seem to understand issues like, I'm a legal aid lawyer and my client's on legal aid so no, I didn't get, like, the crazy bound affidavit with thirty original and certified copies of whatever, because legal aid simply would not pay for that. I could say things like, "Legal aid won't pay for that, Your Honor," and they would understand. . . . [In custody cases, for example,] they won't say things like, "Well, why don't, why don't you drive your child to soccer every other day?" Client doesn't have a car. [They] don't make me say it in open court.

> My old landlord, he helps me out quite a bit and he treats me with
> real, real, real respect and dignity, yeah. He understands some of
> my situation, and you know, he'll help me out. He'll throw me a few
> bucks if I need it, or he says, "If you're stuck for a place for a couple
> of nights, you can come and stay with me."

As these examples suggest, real compassion requires an ability to shift positions—to put oneself in the place of the other and respond not according to one's own needs but in accordance with the real and immediate needs of the other.

Dignity is promoted in relationships between individual and collective actors that are characterized by this kind of *solidarity*. Solidarity means shared identification: seeing other people "as fellow human beings" despite all the trappings of invidious distinction, and realizing "we're all in it together and we have to treat each other that way." Relationships in which there is rapport, familiarity, trust, mutuality, empathy, and reciprocity facilitate the social processes of dignity promotion. Such qualities of solidarity come naturally in social service approaches like peer outreach or peer support where the participants share foundational experiences:

> Because I was homeless, I was in the same predicament with the
> people I'm talking with are or have been. I can relate to it. And I
> try to make people as comfortable as possible. And even when I'm
> interviewing them, if I feel that they are starting to feel a little—that
> I'm being invasive, I bring up that fact, hey, I was homeless before.
> You know, I slept in a car for a year and a half in the park.

Solidarity can be cultivated. One man described the ways in which institutions such as community centers could be used to develop and strengthen solidarity and in this way promote dignity: "Providing program things for people to come together and share the experience. Even when we did [a recent research project], just the whole thing of coming together and the shared experience helped us realize we weren't alone in some of the things that happened. . . . And then plus providing you with that opportunity . . . to do something that might be worthwhile [like art or gardening], you know? And that's what many of these places do."

Dignity promotion and solidarity converge where one's own dignity meets the dignity of others. Ashok Bharti told me:

> You know that [my] dignity is also interlinked with others. If I don't protect the dignity of others, then my dignity also will not be respected. My dignity will also be violated. So protecting dignity means protecting the dignity of everyone. So if I fight for the dignity of others, my dignity ultimately will be served. So everyone has to fight for the dignity of everyone. It can't happen that I fight for the dignity of someone and I lose my dignity. No. It can't happen.

Dignity flourishes in *humane circumstances*: settings where there is calm, ample time and other resources, friendliness, cleanliness, transparency, opportunity, and beauty. Such physical, social, and emotional environments support the dignity of the individuals and groups who frequent them. One mental health care provider described what humane circumstances would look like in the context of a treatment program: "I think that it would be an outpatient program, I mean, in the best-case scenario. In a wonderful, beautiful environment in the community. With money, in terms of like having the space and decorating to feel warm and welcoming . . . lots of opportunity to buy supplies . . . and lots of opportunities for creative endeavors, as well as socialization." A woman who had been homeless drew a similar picture in imagining the ideal environment in which to provide social services. She envisioned a place with comfortable but not lavish furnishings; an excellent arts and crafts program and other activities, including trips into the outdoors; good music playing softly in the background; a wall displaying well-organized information about a wide range of programs and services; and caring counselors trained to aid people in solving problems and accessing resources.

At the broadest level, dignity is promoted in societies structured by a *social order of justice*, a condition that people acknowledged is as yet only aspirational. Dignity, one man said, "relates to justice and justice for all. . . . A lot of it relates to money. So I think if people had, they shouldn't be sparing no expense to make our society a dignified society for all, in terms of providing [income support] services for people or at least providing the education for people, you know, to educate themselves." Another man located dignity enhancement in poverty eradication: "Well, start with addressing poverty. I think poverty is the biggest weapon of mass destruction on the planet. You know, sixty thousand children starve to death every day on the planet. You know, that's—that hurts. So I guess to, yeah, it would be to start at the bottom. . . . The need is greatest at the lower levels, to give people back their dignity." People spoke of human rights regimes as a powerful means of making manifest a social order of justice: "We need human rights protections as the remedy [for dignity violation]. . . . If we work towards a world where we all have dignity . . . then we don't have racism and we don't have poverty and we don't have a lot of other [dignity-violating] things."

Thus, dignity is promoted by a society that supports civic standing by providing adequate income, decent housing, and access to a range of other necessities of life, including education and health care. Such social orders "invest in their citizens," providing the underpinnings of a dignified existence not out of pity or charity, but to answer the demands of fairness and equity.

Just as with vulnerability, antipathy, asymmetry, harshness, and inequality, the contextual conditions of dignity promotion are intertwined and mutually reinforcing. A social order of justice and humane circumstances have a reciprocal relationship with one another and with the other conditions of dignity promotion. Humane circumstances place actors in positions of confidence and compassion. Solidarity commands a social order of justice. A just society provides the tangible elements that constitute a dignified life. Compassion, demonstrated through processes like courtesy, acceptance, and love, creates the humane environments in which dignity thrives. From positions of confidence, individual and collective actors may have the security to interpret gestures in ways that lead their responses to be characterized by resistance rather than shame.

Dignity promotion may be a byproduct of actions and interactions that have nothing to do with dignity per se. As I noted in my description of leveling, an ice cream truck did not visit the campus of the psychiatric hospital to increase patients' dignity (I assume its driver did so to make money by selling ice cream), but the visits nonetheless had the effect of promoting dignity. In many situations, however, dignity promotion is someone's explicit goal, and an actor deploys one or more of the social processes of dignity promotion with intent. I call these deliberate engagements *dignity work*.

This notion of dignity work emerged quite early in the study. Andrew interviewed a young woman who had grown up with a sister who was developmentally disabled. As he and I reviewed the interview and conducted some preliminary analysis, we found many passages in which she was describing how her parents had by their actions impressed on her the need to respect her sister for "who she is as a person." That is, the parents had raised their other children, organized their family life, and made choices about the education and living situation of their disabled daughter with the daughter's dignity uppermost in their minds. They were always working deliberately to promote her dignity. The discovery of dignity work in this interview led us to look for other examples of it, and to begin to ask explicit questions about it during interviews.

People do dignity work for themselves (to promote their own dignity) and for others (to promote the dignity of others). Some types of dignity work are primarily directed at increasing dignity in one's own eyes: some, in the eyes of others. Dignity work may be done by individuals or by collectives—such as organizations, communities, and whole societies—and it may be used to promote the dignity of individuals or of collectives. Many types of dignity work are transitive. Work done to increase the dignity of an individual often promotes the dignity of the group with which the individual identifies. Work done to increase the dignity of the group promotes the dignity of individuals who are members of the group. When people engage in dignity work intended to promote others' dignity, they often find that their own dignity is enhanced as well.

While some types of dignity work are affirmative in nature, others are primarily defensive. Affirmative dignity work seeks to promote human and social dignity or to retain human dignity in situations that deny social dignity. Defensive work is directed at reducing the likelihood of dignity violation or ameliorating the impact of violations that have already taken place.

Finer-grained examination of these broad categories reveals four basic types of dignity work: creating dignity where it is lacking, maintaining existing dignity, protecting dignity that is under threat, and reclaiming dignity that has been lost. Courtesy, empowerment, contribution, discipline, and accomplishment are examples of social processes that may create dignity. Processes like independence, enrichment, authenticity, and love maintain existing dignity. Acceptance, control, transcendence, preparation, avoidance, concealment, presence, and leveling protect dignity that is threatened, while recognition, perseverance, advocacy, support, and resistance may help to reclaim it once it is lost. Affirmative work involving the creation and maintenance of dignity contributes to the development of conditions of confidence, compassion, solidarity, humaneness, and justice. The defensive work of dignity protection and reclamation mitigates conditions of vulnerability, antipathy, asymmetry, harshness, and inequality. In general, the most affirmative types of dignity work, such as courtesy and love, require that some dignity promotion conditions already exist—for example, that an actor have some footing in a position of confidence. Purely defensive dignity work, such as avoidance and concealment, is usually seen under conditions of extreme threat to dignity—often, where an order of inequality is so strong that it leaves individual and collective actors with little ability to do much more than what they need just to survive. Both affirmative and defensive dignity work may meet obstacles. Thus, overcoming barriers to doing dignity work becomes a kind of dignity work in and of itself.

Contradictions and tensions are apparent in dignity work and the social processes of dignity promotion through which it is engaged. In the passages I have quoted, dignity has been seen to be promoted by following rules (accomplishment) and by breaking rules (empowerment), by exercising control (discipline) and by letting go (transcendence), by a belief in the goodness of others (acceptance) and the conviction that such goodness is lacking (avoidance), by being real (authenticity) and by "covering up" (concealment), and by being seen to be like other people (independence) and by being seen to be unique (recognition).

Some of these social processes seem to us more appropriate or healthier than others. When I presented this material to a group of health care providers, they were disturbed that processes like avoidance and concealment, which they saw as counterproductive to dignity, should be used to promote it. The common co-occurrence of resistance and snapping begs the question of whether or not anger and aggression, including the aggression of the strong and powerful directed downwards at the weak and powerless, are also social processes of dignity promotion, or even types of dignity work. I would argue that it depends on context. In some situations, an individual may engage in these belligerent actions and interactions as dignity work; that is, with the intent of promoting his or her own dignity—for example, when the dignity in question is of the "parasitic" type that depends on a "hierarchy of humanness." In other cases, however, these actions and interactions constitute reflexive responses to dignity violation—a kind of consequent "lashing out"—rather than social process used either consciously or unconsciously to promote dignity. Whether intended to be dignity work or not, these oppressive social processes probably do more to decrease human dignity than to increase social dignity.

The *dignity bargain* illustrates some of these contradictions and tensions at work in people's lives. In a dignity bargain, an actor gives up some dignity to get something else she needs, often a material resource. The trade-off is anticipated, assessed, and weighed, and eventually the decision to act is taken in full consciousness of the possible consequences. One woman described these steps to me in the context of her decision to begin accepting several forms of social assistance:

> When these decisions were put in front of me, and I knew my dignity would be taken away, then I thought about it. And I made the decision for myself and I thought, "Now, am I hurting somebody for this? Is this worth the gain of losing my dignity?" And I had to make a conscious decision: Yep. And then I thought, "Am I going to be able to live with my decision? Without carrying it on my back?" Yep. I have to.

Dignity bargainers use dignity as an asset that can be drawn down, with hopes that later it can be renewed. Dignity bargains rely on actors' dignity inventories—their evaluations of the state of their own dignity at the moment and the likely effects of the bargain on their future dignity—both calculations based on their experiences of dignity in the past. Similar assessments are made of the terms of the bargain, including the other actors who are involved and the setting in which the bargain will be negotiated and transacted. Bargains thus are shaped by the context in which they are made. In the example I have quoted, the bureaucracy of poverty and its opportunities and threats determined the speaker's choices. In other bargains, such as those involving family relationships—the decision to leave a marriage, for example—the terms of the bargain will be written by personal and contextual factors like family and community dynamics and cultural or social expectations as exemplified by custom and law. Most dignity bargains contain elements of both affirmative and defensive dignity work.

Through miscalculation, dignity bargains can turn bad, leading to dignity traps. The same woman continued: "Some people will maybe make that decision [to use social services] and can't live with it afterwards. [They] turn to alcohol, turn to drugs, because they really haven't accepted that they could carry that burden of losing your dignity. Some people commit suicide." Dignity bargains can produce "false" dignity. For the woman who concealed her drug use for years, trading authenticity for respectability, the bargain resulted in a simulacrum of dignity that was unsatisfying because she knew it to be false (and dangerous because she always feared being unmasked).

In other cases, a dignity bargain is more beneficial than anticipated:

> So even though I felt the worst thing in the world would be to [live in a subsidized housing complex], that's what I did and it's been the best thing I've ever done. Like instead of taking away what I thought would be my dignity, especially if my family or friends came over, it gave me back [my dignity] because I never had to ask anybody for anything again—because the rent is, you know, geared to income.

The phenomenon of the dignity bargain suggests that while human dignity and the two kinds of social dignity may in some circumstances be promoted through the same social processes, at other times they each require different kinds of work, which can conflict. Independence may ensure a woman's social dignity, but if her basic needs are not fulfilled, her human dignity may remain unrealized. The man who decides to engage in the work of authenticity may reinforce his dignity-of-self at the risk of his dignity-in-relation. There can be no single template for dignity work; it must be exquisitely sensitive to the actors who are engaging in it and the context in which it is engaged.

Dignity promotion affects the same objects that are damaged by dignity violation, helping to create, maintain, protect, and maintain them. Social processes like advocacy and support can work to strengthen the body. The self is sustained and augmented by a panoply of processes, including courtesy, recognition, acceptance, discipline, enrichment, authenticity, love, concealment, and presence. Autonomy is reinforced by empowerment and independence; moral agency is exercised through processes like discipline, perseverance, transcendence, preparation, avoidance, and resistance. Courtesy, recognition, and leveling serve to enhance status, while citizenship is promoted by acceptance, contribution, advocacy, and support. Recognition, authenticity, love, and presence bolster personhood. Directly and indirectly (via their effects on individuals or groups), a people and humanity as a whole may be dignified by any and all of these processes.

The mechanisms linking the social processes of dignity promotion, the conditions that support promotion, the objects of promotion, and the consequences of well-being and flourishing mix the symbolic and the material. Symbolically, dignity promotion strengthens the self. Being treated with dignity "gives you a feeling of, oh, I'm worthy of some, you know, goodness. And then eventually the self-respect will rise." As people become more self-assured, they grow more assertive, refusing to accept the poor treatment they may have endured in the past: "And when they stand up for themselves it's not the angry thing. . . . They have full control. They know they don't deserve that, and they can do it calmly. That gives them even more [dignity]." By enhancing autonomy, moral agency, status, and citizenship, dignity promotion can help to narrow the gap between ideal and actual selves. Shame and its corrosive effects are reduced. When personhood is recognized, one person said, "It's an enormous comfort for people to know that someone else sees that they matter. They might not think they matter; they might think that they matter, but for someone else to see that they matter is enormous. Maybe even life changing." Another asserted, "People can get through the worst things if they're treated as people and they're treated with compassion, with respect, with value."

Materially, the structure and functioning of bodies is supported by the kind of equitable access to necessities like food, housing, health care, and education that define dignified living. Health care facilities and other human services settings that demonstrate dignity-enhancing characteristics are more likely to engage people and to see them return, thus allowing them to benefit from the services offered. When they feel good about who they are, people are motivated to "make a better situation" for themselves. Once people believe that they "matter" to themselves and to others, they are better positioned to make healthy and safe choices, and are able to break some of the personally and socially destructive patterns of the past, such as "giving up" or "lashing out." Just as social epidemiologists have found that disadvantage accumulates over the life span (Marmot and Wilkinson 2006), the stories we heard in our interviews suggest that over time the processes of dignity promotion fill a well of dignity that is both symbolic and material. It can be drawn on as a resource and yet can always be replenished. As the woman I quoted at the beginning of this chapter said, dignity has "gotten me through hardships, through depression, through shame. . . . To hold onto my dignity has really, has kept me going."

At the collective level of a people and humanity, "if you treat people with dignity, you'll get the best out of them." The men and women we interviewed believed that dignity promotion lessens the adverse effects on society of corruption and other kinds of invidious divisions. "It actually is a benefit to society when you, you know, to respect people and to, sort of to think well of somebody instead of thinking negative of somebody." When we recognize and act on the humanity of specific others, we promote their dignity, our own dignity, and the general dignity of all. While a true social order of justice may be a utopia that will always be beyond reach, our individual and collective dignity work—work that is both possible and feasible—draws a virtuous circle, generating the contextual conditions of confidence, compassion, solidarity, and humaneness, and thus creating spaces of justice within the broader orders of inequality that persist, all of which then promotes future enactments of the social processes of dignity promotion.

CHAPTER 5

THE DEMANDS OF DIGNITY

The difficulty comes in trying to spell out the demands of dignity positively, since different people respond indignantly to different actions. The responses are bound up with diverse forms of social life, so that if human dignity is to be a reliable touchstone . . . it should be seen as embedded within these complex forms.
—Evan Simpson (2004)

Thus far, I have focused on the ascriptive and descriptive forms of dignity, examining the literature to understand the theoretical constructions of the grounds of dignity, and using empirical evidence to explore the social processes and contextual conditions that constitute dignity violation and dignity promotion and the consequences of violation and promotion. Dignity also has a prescriptive form. The notion of dignity carries with it obligations of oughts and musts: duties of action and interaction suggestive of what Abraham Edel (1969) called a "normative program," or "an ideal of interpersonal relations and social organization" that can "be woven into concrete areas of human life" (238). Now, I build on the model I have presented in order to look more closely at this aspirational form of dignity—"this more explicitly moral dimension" (Seltser and Miller 1993, 2) of what dignity demands.

There are three such demands. The first is to act (and interact) in ways that may increase, rather than reduce, individual and collective dignity. Dignity is plastic and dynamic—qualities key to my definition of social dignity that I have shown to be at play in the social processes of dignity violation and dignity promotion, including in deliberate dignity work. When dignity promotion is not only a deliberate act, but also a rationalized and institutionalized one, it becomes a *dignity intervention*, a replicable pattern of action and interaction designed to answer dignity's first demand.

The social processes and contextual conditions I have elaborated provide a kind of blueprint for conceptualizing dignity interventions. First, like dignity work more generally, a dignity intervention may be primarily affirmative (focused on promoting dignity) or primarily defensive (focused on reducing dignity violation). Dignity interventions may address processes or conditions, or both. Thus, an affirmative intervention may seek to increase the quality and quantity of the social processes of dignity promotion or it may intercede to create the contextual conditions that structure dignity promotion. A defensive intervention, on the other hand, may focus on decreasing the social processes of violation or on confronting those conditions that determine violation. Both affirmative and defensive interventions may be directed at one or more of the different levels encompassed by the model. An intervention may be aimed at changing the positions of actors or the quality of their relationships (person-level interventions), at changing settings (organizational or system-level interventions), or at changing the social order (societal-level interventions). Finally, a dignity intervention may be directed at a specific object or set of objects. An affirmative, person-level intervention may focus on enhancing feelings of bodily integrity among torture survivors, while a defensive, system-level intervention may aim to reduce policy-based infringements on the citizenship of a people, such as systemic discrimination against a particular ethnic or racial group.

In the first section of this chapter, I offer a number of examples—representative, although not comprehensive—of dignity interventions. I have grouped them by level, beginning with those that address actors and their relationships and moving outward to those that are concerned with transforming the social order. In accordance with this book's emphasis on health, each example pertains to health and social care or to health status more broadly. (One also finds dignity interventions in other arenas: in law enforcement [Lynch 1999], in elementary education [Tuomi 2001], and in foreign policy [Ackerman 2008; Ignatius

2007].) The examples I have selected include interventions that attend specifically to dignity-related problems in health and social care—answers to service users' demands to be treated with dignity in these systems. They also include interventions that seek to moderate the impact of those dignity violations that affect individual and population health—answers to demands to increase individual and collective well-being and flourishing by transforming the social order from one of inequality to one of justice. Some of these examples have been described in the literature in some detail; others are as yet only imagined, but grounded in themes found in my data and in the dignity scholarship more generally. In subsequent sections, I turn to examining the second and then the third demands of dignity.

Any intervention must start with an assessment of the domain for which it is intended. Scholars and advocates have done much to describe the vicissitudes of dignity in the domains of health and social care. Qualitative research has been conducted in a variety of clinical settings—including palliative care, long-term care, acute care, rehabilitation, and pediatrics (Franklin, Ternesdstedt and Nordenfelt 2006; Jacelon 2003; Lundqvist and Nilstun 2007); Mangset et al. 2008; Pleschberger 2007; Stabell and Naden 2006; Street and Kissane 2001; Woogara 2005)—and with a wide range of patient groups—including the elderly, the dying, and persons living with HIV and other chronic illnesses or conditions (Chochinov et al. 2002; Hughes, Davies, and Gudmundsdottir 2008; Soderberg, Lundman, and Norberg 1999; Werner and Malterud 2003). Together, this research has defined and modeled dignity and, especially, identified the intrapersonal and interpersonal pathways through which patients' dignity can be maintained while they are receiving care. Findings from these studies emphasize the importance to dignity of respect and recognition, of choice and control, of psychological and bodily integrity, of privacy, and of comfort and cleanliness.

Quantitative researchers have used large-scale surveys of populations to determine how dignity may be a factor in people's experiences of health care and in their decisions to use health care services (Beach et al. 2005; Blanchard and Lurie 2004; Blendon et al. 2002; Valentine, Darby, and Bonsel 2008). As I noted in Chapter 3, these studies have established that people value dignity in health care and that dignity has tangible consequences for service utilization.

The nursing profession has been particularly committed to researching dignity in practice. In article after article, nurse-researchers have reviewed what is known about dignity and explored the implications of this knowledge for care provision (e.g., Birrell, Thomas, and Jones 2006; Coventry 2006; Griffin-Heslin 2005; Jacelon et al. 2004; Jacobs 2000, 2001; Mairis 1994; Matiti, Cotrel-Gibbons, and Teasdale 2007; Milton 2008; Shotton and Seedhouse 1998; Soderberg, Gilje, and Norberg 1997). A review of this theoretical, empirical, and practical work concluded that nurses could best promote dignity for their patients by paying attention to four facets of care: the physical environment in which care is provided, including the cleanliness of the accommodations and the privacy available; the attitudes and behavior of staff who interact with patients, including the forms of address they use when speaking to patients; the culture of care, including cultural competence among the staff and the existence of advocacy services in the institution; and, finally, the manner in which specific care activities—such as feeding and toileting—are performed (Gallagher et al. 2008).

In health and social care, then, dignity has been conceptualized largely as "transactional" (Chochinov 2003, 307), arising at the confluence of subjective experience and objective conditions (George 1998). It is a psychosocial property that may be created or destroyed in interactions between providers and patients or, more broadly, in the spaces of practice and policy where patient populations, provider groups, and the structures and processes of the health care system intersect. The uses of dignity in health care have been highly instrumental, aimed at "furnishing a direction for the achievement of purposes and the solution of problems" (Edel 1969, 238).

While a few authors have questioned the usefulness of dignity as a guiding concept in health care (for example, Wainwright and Gallagher [2008] have suggested that "an appeal to respect" [53] might be more effective), the idea appears to have generated little controversy. In practice, however, there are many barriers to dignity in health and social care. I have characterized these barriers as resulting from a series of tensions: the opposition between needs and resources, privacy and exposure, crisis and routine, care and production, autonomy and authority, experience and expertise, treatment and punishment, and rhetoric and reality. Together, these tensions describe an institution in which dignity is thwarted by the multiple scarcities (including those scarcities of time and empathy) provoked by what one person I spoke to called "economic thinking," by enduring asymmetries of prestige and power, and by narrow technocratic definitions of quality and accountability that result in policies and procedures that are demeaning for both the users and the providers of care (Jacobson 2009b). The rhetoric of dignity is pervasive in health and social care—witness the plethora of government white papers and organizational mission statements that wield the term—but, as we have seen, the reality is something very different.

In our discussions with people who are users and providers of health and social services, we found that they were acutely aware of the structural determinants of dignity in health and social care. They were able to make connections between the tensions I have described and the health and social care services with which they interacted. Even in the midst of describing incidents of indifference and dismissal perpetrated by doctors and other health care providers, people often stopped to note the pressures of time built into Canada's fee-for-service system of physician reimbursement or indicated their awareness of the status hierarchies that determine relations between different occupational groups in health and social care settings. (Interestingly, even very hard-done-by clients were sensitive to the ways in which these structural factors are as destructive to the dignity of service providers as they are to the dignity of service users. As one man mused while talking about the behavior of income support bureaucrats who had offended his dignity, "Would I feel very dignified working for a system that does not allow people to live properly?")

Of particular interest in these conversations was the picture that emerged of the component parts of the broad institution of health and social care. For the users of services, the most salient elements of health and social care are the staff with whom they interact when accessing services, the nature of the services on offer (e.g., medical care, income support, housing), and the rules of the organizations that are in the business of providing these services. Providers sketched a similar (though perhaps somewhat more detailed) typology, describing an institution that is constituted by individual providers and clients, by jobs, by organizations, and by an overarching system of government oversight and regulation. Taken together, these catalogs of parts provide a map to possible points of dignity intervention.

The knowledge, attitudes, and behaviors of both service providers and clients are mentioned again and again as important to realizing dignity in health and social care. Such knowledge, attitudes, and behaviors reside at the first level of conditions in my model—that is, the level at which dignity encounters are structured by the positions of these individual and collective actors and the relationships between them. Dignity is enhanced when providers and clients are in positions of confidence and compassion and when their relationships are characterized by solidarity; it is threatened when they are in positions of vulnerability and antipathy and their relationships are asymmetrical.

Both users and providers of health and social services spoke of the qualities of providers that indicated positions of compassion. Clients described such providers as attentive, trustworthy, sensitive, and empathic. They are able to "relate" to their clients' difficulties (rather than being shocked or repulsed by them) and actively seek to "play down" their prestige and authority, in this way leveling asymmetry and starting to forge relationships based on solidarity. (Providers in positions of antipathy demonstrate contempt toward their clients and maximize asymmetry in their relationships by attempting to wield absolute control over their clients' lives.) According to clients and to providers themselves, these qualities are either inborn as a matter of temperament or achieved through professional training or, more likely, life experience.

The person-level dignity interventions suggested included better screening of people seeking work in human services and more (and better) training focused on skills such as listening and building trust. Shared experience emerged as particularly important to the leveling of asymmetry and the development of solidarity. Both clients and providers suggested it would be fruitful to foster this characteristic, either by recruiting providers from among client communities or by finding ways to emphasize what providers and clients may hold in common. A mental health services worker suggested that with every client interaction, providers learn ask themselves one simple question: "If my mother came to this service, would I want her to be treated this way?"

The literature contains descriptions of several interventions designed to address the dignity-related knowledge, attitudes, and behaviors of health and social care providers. These interventions tend to mix the defensive and the affirmative, seeking both to reduce providers' engagement in dignity violation and to increase their enactment of the social processes of dignity promotion. Milika Matiti, Elizabeth Cotrel-Gibbons, and Kevin Teasdale (2007) focus on "rais[ing] awareness of patient dignity by encouraging nurses to reflect on the concept and ensure they have the knowledge, skills and an appropriate attitude to support it" (46). Their intervention asks nurses to explore what dignity means to them in their own lives, then to turn that raised consciousness to their practice, using techniques like SWOT (strengths, weaknesses, opportunities, and threats) analysis to assess their abilities to recognize and address the dignity needs of their patients. Harvey Max Chochinov (2007) has published a similar set of self-reflective exercises for physicians; his intervention includes a primer on attitude and behavior that is particularly concerned with heightening physician compassion and facilitating a dignity-promoting communication style. Annie Parsons and Claire Hooker (2010) have argued that providers should attain a "narrative competence" that allows them to elicit and respond to patients' stories, in this way reinforcing dignity-of-self. The most recent edition of the bible of nursing care planning features a care plan for the nursing diagnosis of "risk for compromised dignity" (Ackley and Ladwig 2008). It provides guidance to nurses in recognizing the risk factors for compromised patient dignity (things like "cultural incongruity" and "stigmatized label") and suggests steps nurses can take to maintain patients' dignity and increase their hope. *Educating for Dignity* (c. 2004), a product of the Dignity and Older Europeans study (Calnan, Badcott, and Woolhead 2006; Tadd and Calnan 2009; Woolhead et al. 2006), focuses on the dignity of older people in health and social care, using the theoretical model of dignity developed by the study investigators to explore the social context of old age and the risks to dignity faced by elderly people who are using care services. This manual for educational intervention, designed for use in group or workshop settings, engages providers in discussions of the meaning of dignity and the practice of dignity-supporting care. Unlike the other provider-focused interventions I have described, it seeks to get people to reflect on the social and cultural factors that affect dignity in old age, as well as the structural factors that underpin frontline workers' ability (or inability) to deliver dignity-promoting care.

The positions of client actors in health and social care also present a possible point of intervention. Care plans and many other published interventions help providers recognize particular vulnerabilities and act in the moment to mitigate them—for example, by using empathic language or by closing bed curtains. The literature contains other interventions designed to address the vulnerability of individuals who are experiencing particular health conditions or facing a period of institutional care. These interventions are largely affirmative in their approach, aiming to move people into positions of confidence. Dignity therapy, a psychotherapeutic approach developed by psychiatrist Harvey Max Chochinov and his colleagues (Chochinov 2002, 2007; Chochinov et al. 2002) seeks to help individuals who are terminally ill create their own legacies, in this way "bolstering their sense of meaning, purpose and dignity" (Chochinov 2007, 187). (At this writing, there are two randomized controlled trials of dignity therapy in progress that are designed to assess the feasibility, acceptability, and effectiveness of the technique.)

A potential intervention is suggested by Milika Matiti and Gillian Trorey's (2004) concept of *perceptual adjustment*: "A psychological preparation for the potential violation of dignity in a hospital situation" in which "a patient forecasts the potential indignities that he or she expects to suffer when in hospital, mentally analyses the situation and adjusts to a level that he or she feels comfortable enough to accept" (741). Perceptual adjustment is sensitive to changing conditions. "Individual patients each have their own expectations with regard to their dignity and these perceptions may change in relation to the level of health" (Matiti and Trorey 2008, 2716). That is, a very sick person may be less likely to perceive insults to her dignity, or more likely to accept such insults, than a person who is almost well. Perceptual adjustment, which is somewhat similar to the concept of the dignity bargain that I have described, thus holds promise as the core of an intervention designed to assess and inform patient expectations in order to ensure an alignment between these expectations, a patient's health status, and the care provided.

Most of the providers I interviewed admitted that some clients are harder than others to treat with dignity. They indicated that most difficult are those clients who are physically violent or who threaten violence and those who are offensive (individuals who use racial slurs or who "violate boundaries" by yelling at providers and other staff). Patients who "sabotage" their own treatment by ignoring advice, breaking agreements, or just not showing up, and, as I noted earlier, those who guard their rights so zealously that they put providers on the defensive are also hard to treat with dignity. Arguably, many of these behaviors represent forms of dignity work engaged in response to previous dignity violations, and such clients are in the positions of greatest vulnerability to future violations.

Rather than relying on defensive interventions such as care plans once a threat to dignity has been identified, a more effective strategy might involve longer term and more ambitious affirmative approaches to building up the dignity resources held by these clients, thus shifting them into positions of confidence. The men and women we interviewed suggested that dignity resources usually originate in childhood, but that when family dysfunction or other disruptions interfere with their development, they can be obtained later in life. Many of the social processes of dignity promotion I described in Chapter 4 might be marshaled for such interventions. Indeed, several of the people we spoke with used various forms of therapy and skill building (like gender-based assertiveness training), as well as creativity and spirituality, in just this way.

In her book *Respect*, Sara Lawrence-Lightfoot (1999) sketched detailed portraits of six people, including two health care providers, who were expert at enacting respect in their work. Lawrence-Lightfoot's focus was on the autobiographies of the individuals she profiled and the qualities of their actions and interactions at work, but she also looked at the ways in which her subjects' approaches shaped and were shaped by their workplace environments. Similarly, the model I have described situates dignity. The positions and relationships of providers and clients cannot be separated from the conditions of their settings; dignity-related knowledge, attitudes, and behaviors are dependent on the give and take between individuals and the structures in which they operate. Dignity interventions in health and social care therefore must address not just persons, but also organizations and systems.

Both clients and providers described multiple challenges to dignity in health and social care that reside at the organizational and system levels. Clients spoke of the rigid and sometimes opaque and arbitrarily applied rules and regulations that seek to homogenize them, of the trials and tribulations inherent in the "runaround," and of the paucity and poor quality of many of the services they need. Providers referenced jobs that are structured so as to make them feel surveilled, distrusted, isolated, and sometimes even abused, as well as always frantic with busyness; workplace cultures that lack dignity-oriented leadership, the time and space to think about dignity, and even a language with which to discuss it; and a system that is apparently concerned with bureaucratic processes of standardization and documentation above all else. These factors come together in what both clients and providers pointed to as the organizational and systemic disincentives to complaint that conspire to make dignity violation invisible. As one provider said:

If you're making a complaint about somebody, it usually has to be very clear because it's difficult to make a—it's a difficult process to make a complaint. . . . It's easier when someone made a very clear mistake . . . whereas dignity is so—it's so subjective and hard to describe and we're not, you know, so well languaged in [talking about it]. It's much harder to say, "You did something wrong," and they could say, "No, I didn't," you know. "Tell me exactly what I did wrong." And it's just harder to explain the impact or the actual initial problem.

The organizational interventions suggested by the men and women we spoke to were directed at moving service provision environments away from these harsh circumstances and toward circumstances that were more humane. They wanted to see changes in physical environments—more attention to the aesthetics of place, more egalitarian uses of space. They urged the establishment of practices to provide more information and to sustain clearer lines of communication. They called for the implementation of activities that give service users a voice, such as patient advocacy groups or meaningful assessments of client satisfaction. Finally, a number of service providers argued that organizations should support collective reflection among their personnel: "We need to make it a point to discuss dignity, both for ourselves internally and for those that we serve. . . . Work needs to be done around identifying and making it very clear for people. People know what dignity is, but I think more discussions need to take place around its value and its impact and how fragile dignity is, and yet how brilliant it is."

Both clients and providers perceived service provision organizations that use what they described as a social justice model (which I understand as a framework that sees individuals' problems as microcosms of societal injustices and views working toward social change as equal in importance to providing individual treatment) as tending to be more conducive to dignity. Clients found such organizations to be flexible and transparent in their policies and procedures: they provided services where clients found themselves, rather than requiring them to make office visits; they operated on a drop-in basis instead of by appointment; and they allowed clients to begin receiving services before completing the formalities (and intrusions) of intake. A number of providers noted that working for social justice-oriented agencies promoted their own dignity because they felt in sync with their organizations' missions and were more likely to share important values and commitments with their colleagues. The interventions envisioned, then, sought to develop cultures within other services that emulated the salient features of these enterprises—especially their creative and transgressive ability to challenge the status quo or break the rules by engaging in what Cathy Crowe described as "practice out of the box."

Organizations that provide health and social care services are also workplaces. To promote worker dignity, employees argued, service provision agencies should strive to maintain adequate resources (including time and support for self-care), nonautocratic decision-making processes, some task variety, respect for workers' skills, and the autonomy for workers to do their jobs as they see fit in order to best serve their clients. The importance of these qualities is reinforced by dignity scholarship produced by sociologists of work, which, although not drawn specifically from the health domain, suggests ways in which health and social care workplaces might be organized so as to promote the dignity of their staff (and thus, by transitive extension, the people who use their services.)

In his synthesis of dignity at work across a number of industries,

Randy Hodson (2001) found that workers' dignity is threatened by mismanagement and abusive behavior (displayed by managers against employees or among co-workers), by overwork, by limited autonomy, and by the contradictions of employee involvement—claims to value worker participation that are in fact cynical attempts to increase worker productivity (all situations that would be very familiar to the health and social care workers I interviewed). Workers' dignity is promoted by "organizational cultures of respect" (232): environments that foster positive relations between management and staff, a livable pace of work, work processes that allow for creativity and meaning, and authentic forms of worker agency. Similarly, Paula M. Rayman (2001) reported that dignity-enhancing workplaces feature continual learning, meaningful worker participation, and the implementation of policies that support the social ties that connect workers to one another and to their families and communities. Together, these studies point to the dignity that can be found by designing health and social care workplaces so that they support frontline care workers' education and skill building, encourage their autonomy, and strengthen their social connections.

At the system level, the people I interviewed wanted to see imaginative and innovative interventions that improved service access, coordination, and quality for the most vulnerable individuals and groups, such as people who are homeless and mentally ill. One outreach worker said:

> [These people] need a system that isn't so difficult to access. A lot of clients, you know, who are living on the street or are homeless or are chronically on the verge of homelessness don't necessarily have the wherewithal to go and see a doctor and follow up and go and see a psychiatrist and take their meds and follow through on that.... We need other ways, other points of access to the health care system. For example, the shelters.... There are more and more doctors who are based at shelters and seeing clients at shelters, so that kind of access I think is needed.... We need to think outside the box in terms of how to deliver that to these individuals.

A man who was living in a shelter had similar ideas about what was needed:

Everything's there if you want it, you know what I mean? They have, they have staff for mental health, they have [staff] for housing. It's all right there on site so you don't have to go anywhere to, to get anything, you know what I mean? And with medical and this and that, whatever. And they also, when you first get that interview and they ask you all the questions to see what you need and what they, what they can help you with and stuff like that, yeah.

In addition, there were suggestions that systems reduce the size of frontline workers' case loads to allow more individualized care and that they make room for new categories of personnel, like patient navigators who could help people find their way through the confusing labyrinths of the system. Frustrated with the provincially mandated outcome measures her mental health services agency was forced to track, one social worker described an alternative set of dignity-oriented indicators that might be used to assess her organization's work: "Is the person able to trust her intuition?" "Is the person considering the future?" "Is the person engaged with the world?" "Is the person able to advocate for himself?"

Both clients and providers urged more systemic support for nontraditional modes of service provision—such as peer support and harm reduction—that advance humane circumstances and animate solidarity. Peer support, Shawn Lauzon said, provides its participants with the "ongoing support, the dialogue, the sharing of experiences, so that it allows a person to say, 'Yeah, OK, so that's who I am' . . . and I think it's in that context that that's where a person starts thinking about what happens for them, what they still need, what they can still do to get what they need . . . in order to live their productive lives, their, their dignified lives." Harm reduction, a social worker noted, is "a method of respecting a person's dignity by giving them, giving them some sense of control over what's going on in their lives versus saying, 'We're not going to provide this service to you unless you can be completely abstinent.'" Harm reduction respects "people's choices" and recognizes "where people are at instead of forcing them to be, you know, something you'd like them to be." Indeed, recent research suggests that these approaches can be highly effective at promoting the dignity of the people who participate in them (Ben-Ishai 2012; Jacobson and Dewa 2009).

A novel form of systemic intervention proposed by several of the people I interviewed was to institute a policy of "reality checking." Based on the widely held belief that, as one woman I quoted earlier said, "the higher you go, the smaller the 'd' in dignity," reality checking meant requiring powerful people to experience the positions of those over whom they wield their power. Service providers should have to walk in their clients' shoes, even if just for a short while. Agency administrators should have to spend time working on the front lines of service provision. Politicians should have to apply to use the services affected by their decisions. As a woman who was receiving disability support said of the government officials whose policy choices determined many facets of her daily life:

> [I would tell them] to get down in the trenches and live there for a while . . . to experience and to taste what reality is, that's probably what I would say . . . and I don't mean just for a day, have anybody in any seat of power to take that cloak off, and get down and live with the common folk, make it mandatory, you know, and live like the rest of us for a while and understand what it's like.

Published descriptions of organizational-level dignity interventions for health and social care focus on program planning and service delivery, care guidelines and benchmarks, and dignity-oriented accountability structures. While some of these interventions use the language of dignity directly, others frame it using component or related concepts like empowerment or health equity. Jan E. Thomas (2000) examined feminist women's health centers and their strategies for empowering both service users and service providers. She found that such centers create environments of dignity and respect by providing clients with education and information and by breaking down traditional institutional barriers through, for example, making their physical and social environments welcoming and increasing average appointment time. A number of reports have suggested ways in which hospitals might implement (Betancourt et al. 2009) and monitor (Centre for Research on Inner City Health 2009) policies and practices designed to reduce health disparities and promote health equity among populations vulnerable to discrimination and other deprivations of access and outcome.

Interventions designed to promote dignity at the level of health systems use similar ideas as applied to system design and accountability. In a document containing recommendations aimed at fostering equity in Ontario's provincial health care system, Bob Gardner (2008) provided guidelines for how system planners might promote dignity by prioritizing the most marginalized members of society in their planning processes: focus on the social determinants of health, target the poorest neighborhoods and demographic groups, and always use equity as a lens to assess the impact of all decisions. Paula Braveman and Sofia Gruskin (2003) similarly emphasized the social determinants of health in their recommendations for promoting equity in health systems. Their framework addressed issues of planning and monitoring, with particular attention to preventive care and health care financing. They also highlighted the need to address health equity concerns in policy sectors outside of health.

In the model of dignity I have described, positions, relationships, and settings are always mutually reinforcing. Because of this interdependence, dignity interventions at the person, organizational, and system levels must also be intertwined, if not practically, at least conceptually. (That is, although a person-level intervention may not engage system-level conditions directly, it must be designed and implemented with knowledge of those conditions.) The "Dignity in Care" campaign in the United Kingdom is an example of a dignity intervention that in its design and implementation attempts to integrate all three levels.

"Dignity in Care" focuses on the dignity of older people in systems of health and social care. Initiated in the late 1990s by a British advocacy group called Help the Aged, it has been taken up and elaborated by other nongovernmental organizations and by various governmental advisory and oversight bodies in a campaign known as the "Dignity in Care Challenge." Campaign participants have undertaken empirical research and policy analysis, issuing a number of reports that vividly describe threats to the dignity of elderly people who are users of health and social care services. Using these findings, the campaign has provoked further government investigations and the funding and implementation of a multipronged strategy to address the problems identified. Among the components of this strategy are continued efforts at raising public awareness; educational programming for health and social care providers, including the production of instructional materials; network development; personnel deployment ("dignity champions" and the controversial "dignity nurses"); organizational and system-level guidelines, standards, and benchmarks; surveys and assessments; a series of specific policy recommendations; and tools for monitoring and evaluating the impact of these interventions (Bates 2008; Birrell, Thomas, and Jones 2006; Butler 2006; Healthcare Commission 2007; Jones and Aranda 2009; Levenson 2007; Magee, Parsons, and Askham 2008; Sandler 2006).

The campaign has sought to engage a broad range of domains of action and interaction. Help the Aged has argued for a focus on matters of communication, privacy, self-determination and autonomy, direct payments, food and nutrition, pain and symptom control, personal hygiene, personal care and home help, death with dignity, and social inclusion (Bates 2008; Levenson 2007). In their work, the Commission for Healthcare Audit and Inspection has looked at a number of Help the Aged's domains, but also added assessments of patient involvement, dementia and confusion, workforce, leadership, complaints, and community partnerships (Healthcare Commission 2007). Other campaign participants have introduced the legal domains of abuse, complaint, and redress (Butler 2006).

"No standard working definition for dignity" has emerged from the campaign (Healthcare Commission 2007, 15). Without a single definition, campaign participants have been free to proffer meanings that best serve their aims. Advocacy organizations have promoted a conceptualization of dignity that blends elements of both human and social dignity (Butler 2006; Levenson 2007), as reflected in Help the Aged's dignity principles:

- Dignity in care is inseparable from the wider context of dignity as a whole.
- Dignity is about treating people as individuals.
- Dignity is not just about physical care.
- Dignity thrives in the context of equal power relationships.
- Dignity must be actively promoted.
- Dignity is more than the sum of its parts. (Levenson 2007, 13)

Standard setting and measurement have also been used as proxies for definition. Thus, the Commission for Healthcare Audit and Inspection looks to social dignity phenomena like staff behavior and the presence or absence of organizational "systems" for safeguarding dignity (Healthcare Commission 2007). A set of indicators developed to assess Help the Aged's dignity domains similarly focuses on broad themes of staff attitudes, facilities, choice, and control as these are manifested in each domain (Magee, Parsons, and Askham 2008).

The breadth of domains claimed by the campaign and its definitional flexibility have allowed for the development of a similarly broad collection of interventions. Exhortatory and educational interventions have addressed frontline providers, administrators, and the general public, seeking to build awareness of dignity issues and increase capacity among the care workforce to deal with these issues. Specific tools have been designed to guide frontline providers' behaviors in areas like privacy and to benchmark the dignity component of care quality in service provision. These dignity-related best practices and standards also have aimed to change administrative and organizational procedures and practices, while the development of regulatory structures and the invocation of legal authority are designed to influence systemic policy.

Critics of the campaign as it is actually being implemented, however, fault its failure to move much beyond the individual level of provider knowledge, attitude, and behavior (Jones and Aranda 2009; Aranda and Jones 2010). Pointing to the kinds of structural constraints I have already described in health care settings, their critiques suggest the need for the campaign to promote a more politically sophisticated and socially situated understanding of dignity and to make organizations and systems, rather than individuals, the targets of change.

In the model of dignity I have presented, dignity is more easily violated under a social order of inequality that perpetuates itself through systems of hierarchy, dispossession, and oppression. When asked to talk about the underlying causes of dignity violation in their own lives, the men and women we interviewed consistently pointed to social order phenomena like the lack of educational opportunity, unemployment, unaffordable housing, poverty, and prejudice and discrimination. The literature on the social determinants of population health focuses on such phenomena writ large (Commission on the Social Determinants of Health 2008; Marmot and Wilkinson 2006). Those who study local and global health inequities and those who organize to fight them attribute the widespread damage wrought by these forms of structural violence to globalization and, in particular, to the spread of a neoliberal political ideology that values profits over people (Birn 2009; Chapman 2009; Farmer 2005; People's Health Movement 2000; Raphael 2004; Sharma and Bharti 2005). Such manifestations of hierarchy, dispossession, and oppression may best be addressed using human rights theory and practice.

Modern human rights were codified in the years immediately following the Second World War when, prompted by the Holocaust, representatives of the United Nations member countries, led by Eleanor Roosevelt, sought to devise a "an instrument of ordering international relations" (Arieli 2002, 3) based on such "universal" values as liberty, equality, and unity (Morsink 1999). The product of their efforts, the Universal Declaration of Human Rights (1948), consists of thirty articles that delineate a set of rights encompassing what Stephen Marks (2003) described as "rights of autonomous action," such as civil rights; "rights of social interaction," such as the rights to education and civic participation; and "rights of existence," such as the rights to life and health. Together with its follow-up documents, the International Covenant on Civil and Political Rights (1966) and the International Covenant on Economic, Social, and Cultural Rights (1966), which provide more detailed accounts of these rights (and are legally binding on the countries that have ratified them), the declaration speaks to the relationship between the individual and the state, detailing "what governments *can* do *to* us, *cannot* do *to* us, and *should* do *for* us" (Gruskin and Tarantola 2000, 4; emphases in the original).

Dignity is a fundamental need for all human beings (Ignatieff 1984) and thus is woven into the fabric of human rights. The preamble of the Universal Declaration begins by recognizing the "inherent dignity . . . of all members of the human family" and "the dignity and worth of the human person," while the preambular language of both International Covenants states that the rights inscribed "derive from the inherent dignity of the human person." Philosophers, political theorists, and legal scholars concerned with human rights have emphasized this grounding of human rights in dignity (Hailer and Ritschl 1996; Meeks

1984; Schachter 1983), arguing that dignity is antecedent, not consequent to human rights (Gewirth 1992); that dignity represents "a right to rights" (Klein 2002, 147); that the capacity to make claims to rights is a manifestation of dignity (Feinberg 1970; Meyer 1989); that dignity cannot be "realized in action" without human rights (Meeks 1984, xi); and that human rights law is a codification of dignity (Paust 1984). Deryck Beyleveld and Roger Brownsword (2001) explained the logic linking dignity to human rights: "That each and every human being has inherent *dignity*; that it is this *inherent* dignity that grounds (or accounts for) the possession of human rights (it is from such inherent dignity that such rights are *derived*); that these are *inalienable* rights; and that, because all humans have dignity, they hold these rights *equally*" (13; emphases in the original).

Although there has been some criticism of dignity in the human rights arena—that its meaning is not clear (Feldman 2000; Zhang 2000) and that it is overly psychological and individualistic in orientation and thus downplays the obligations of governments to populations (Liebenberg 2005)—in the main, the use of dignity in human rights appears to have been widely accepted (Becker 2001). There has been little discussion of the ground of dignity (an exception being that of Michael Ignatieff [2001], who argued that the ground of dignity in human rights should be agency), and thus little opportunity to dismiss it as reflective of an overly restrictive ideological perspective. (This lack of controversy is very likely to have been, at least in part, the result of a decision by the Universal Declaration's drafters to omit any attribution of the origins of dignity or the other "universal" values they championed—in particular to avoid all intimations of a religious ground—to maintain the acceptability of the document to a diverse audience [Baker 2001; Dicke 2002; Morsink 1999].) Rather, the focus has been on the implications of dignity for the enactment of human rights principles.

The growth of the human rights perspective has had the effect of "reconfigur[ing] our socially constituted understanding of who is fully human and therefore possesses all of the dignity and legal rights accorded to those already recognized as full human beings" (Yamin 2009, 5). Acceptance of the "worth of the human person" as a guiding value in human rights invokes claims to "a basic respect . . . and a basically dignified existence" (Paust 1984, 167) for all human beings. These claims are both positive in nature (requiring affirmative action or intervention) and negative (requiring the practice of noninterference). Philosophers, legal scholars, and political scientists who have engaged dignity theoretically are uniform in their assertion that "the demands of dignity impose a minimum standard of decent treatment for every individual" (Goodin 1981, 97). Indeed, the connection between dignity and human rights is so strong that failures to meet the expectations created by widespread knowledge of the existence of these rights may lead to a kind of individual and collective humiliation (Lindner 2006).

Those men and women I interviewed who were researchers, practitioners, or activists engaged in the work of promoting human rights believed that, despite some set-backs, over time the trajectory of dignity in the world generally has been an upward one. The World Dignity Forum's Ashok Bharti said, "I am very optimistic. This history of the world indicates with every day passing dignity is becoming the major concern of the human civilization. You know, at the time of the, I mean, look at the history. There was the slaves. There was the serfs. We have the struggle against [those] systems. And the dignity of the human beings is increasing and indeed becoming equal and paramount. So I'm very optimistic about it."

Human rights claims based on dignity are relevant to collectives, at the societal level, but also pertain to individuals. Such claims rest on an abstraction, but to be meaningful "must address the actual lived experience of any and all individuals in quite different circumstances" (Fischlin and Nandorfy 2007). One very fruitful domain for claims based on the application of human rights principles has been in public health.

The health and human rights approach was catalyzed by a convergence of health and politics in the late twentieth century, especially by the HIV epidemic, continuing controversy over women's reproductive health issues, and politically motivated mass violence such as the Rwandan genocide (Gruskin and Tarantola 2000). Such population health–related phenomena revealed to some observers the limitations of current theory and practice in public health. Jonathan Mann, one of the founders of the health and human rights movement, described these limitations: "First, public health has lacked a conceptual framework for identifying and analyzing the societal factors that represent the 'conditions in which people can be healthy.' Second, a related problem: public health lacks a vocabulary with which to speak about and identify commonalities among health problems experienced by very different populations. Third, there is no consensus about the nature or direction of societal change that would be necessary to address the societal conditions involved" (1997, 8). Human rights concepts and language could, he argued, address all three of these deficits.

Application of human rights ideas to public health scholarship and practice resulted in an approach with three main foci: how health policies, programs, and practices may impinge upon or promote human rights, how human rights violations affect health, and, building on an understanding of these two reciprocal relationships, how the "promotion and protection of human rights and promotion and protection of health are fundamentally linked" (Mann et al. 1999, 11). In keeping with other modern frameworks in public health, the health and human rights approach reaches beyond the biomedical model and its emphasis on individual behavior and clinical care, using a broad definition of health as holistic well-being and focusing on the social determinants of population health. The approach has moved "toward a more expansive understanding of the relationships between human health, medicine and the environment, socioeconomic and civil and political rights, and public health initiatives and human rights" (Knowles 2001, 260). That is, its innovation has been to see the promotion, protection, and fulfillment of the interdependent civil, political, economic, social, and cultural rights inscribed in the Universal Declaration of Human Rights (or failures to promote, protect, and fulfill these rights) as determinants of individual and collective health.

Dignity is used in several ways in the health and human rights movement. Because dignity is understood to be the basis of all human rights, positive and negative claims to "basic respect . . . and a basically dignified existence" are themselves conceptualized as determinants of health (Marks 2003). Paul Farmer (2005) described the phenomenon of structural violence as "a broad rubric that includes a host of offensives against human dignity," such as "extreme and relative poverty" and "social inequalities ranging from racism to gender inequality" (8). Dignity is also portrayed in the health and human rights literature as dependent on health; good health is "a precondition for the capacity to realize and enjoy human rights and dignity" (Mann et al. 1999, 18). (It follows, then, that dignity is at greater risk under conditions of poor health.) Finally, as I explored in Chapter 3, the subjective experience of dignity violation is posited to be a biopsychosocial mechanism linking social conditions and health: human rights violations, in addition to being moral wrongs, are also stressors that affect individual and collective health status through the damage they inflict on dignity. Via dignity, rights violations trigger a panoply of emotional, psychological, physical, behavioral, and social harms that lower resistance and increase susceptibility to disease and ill health (Chilton 2006; Mann 1998).

These uses construe dignity as a property of the environment, of action and interaction, and a condition of experience that can be inventoried, ordered, measured, and then made the target of intervention. Indeed, Jonathan Mann and his colleagues (1999) noted that "a coherent vocabulary and framework to categorize dignity and many forms of dignity violation are lacking" and called for research leading to "a taxonomy and an epidemiology of violations of dignity" (15). In health and human rights, then, dignity's main function is as a risk factor or a protective factor, a linchpin in the casual linkage between the promotion and protection of human rights and the promotion and protection of health.

Dignity's first demand is articulated in claims based on human rights principles. Dieter Birnbacher (1996) listed the "minimal rights" that should characterize oft-cited ideals of basic respect and dignified existence: "(1) Provision of the biologically necessary means of existence, (2) freedom from strong and continued pain, (3) minimal liberty, (4) minimal self-respect" (110). Oscar Schachter (1983) argued that dignity implies "a high priority should be accorded in political, social and legal arrangements to individual choices in such matters as beliefs, way of life, attitudes and the conduct of public affairs" (849) and should prompt "recognition of a minimal concept of distributive justice that would require satisfaction of the essential needs of everyone" (851). David Feldman (1999) singled out prevention of discrimination against individuals and groups as key to dignity. In their comprehensive framework for an "international law of human dignity," Myres S. McDougal, Harold D. Lasswell, and Lung-chu Chen (1980) envisioned the implementation of multiple "human dignity values": "Respect—freedom of choice, equality, and recognition; power—making and influencing community decisions; enlightenment—gathering, processing, and disseminating information and knowledge; well-being—safety, health, and comfort; wealth—production, distribution, and consumption of goods and services, control of resources; skill—acquisition and exercise of capabilities in vocations, professions, and the arts; affection—intimacy, friendship, loyalty, positive sentiments; rectitude—participation in forming and applying norms of responsible conduct" (85).

A general list of the tangible resources that might ensure a dignified existence may be found in the International Covenant on Economic, Social, and Cultural Rights (1966). They include "adequate food, clothing and housing" and "the continuous improvement of living conditions" (Article 11); employment under "just and favourable conditions," including the receipt of fair wages (Articles 6–8); education, including primary education that is "compulsory and available free to all" (Articles 13–14); child protection (Article 10); participation in cultural life (Article 15); and "the highest attainable standard of physical and mental health," including access to health services (Article 12). Martha Nussbaum (2000) sought to elucidate "the bare minimum of what respect for human dignity requires" (5) for each person in a society to "live really humanly" (74). She identified a list of "capabilities," underpinnings that allow individuals "to do and to be," that includes life, health, imagination, practical reason, affiliation, and control over one's political and material environment. In the field of international development, Charles Omondi Oyaya and Dan C. O. Kaseje (2001) generated a list of the "essential elements of dignified living," which include food security, land ownership, education, income, housing, health care access, access to water and sanitation, access to information, institutionalization of action, a sense of belonging, and peace and security. Thus, dignity implies a positive right of access to the resources necessary for well-being and flourishing, as well as a negative right to protection from that which may threaten well-being or deny flourishing.

Human rights principles may be used to realize a dignity-based health policy by suggesting interventions that target health and social care organization or systems. In the United Kingdom, the Equality and Human Rights Group (2008) developed a framework for implementing the key human rights values of fairness, respect, equality, dignity, and autonomy in health and social care. Their framework supports a process that begins with human rights education, facilitates understanding of the practical utility of applying human rights in health and social care, and then leads organizations to ways in which they might operationalize rights in their care planning and service delivery. Among the case studies presented in the group's materials are several health care trusts that have put human rights principles like nondiscrimination, empowerment, and participation to work in their planning and accountability practices. "General Comment 14: The Right to the Highest Attainable Standard of Health" (Committee on Economic, Social and Cultural Rights 2000) sets out a rights-based framework for health systems that is constituted by four dignity-related aspirations: availability, accessibility, acceptability, and quality. Gunilla Backman and her co-authors (2008) proposed a set of indicators that may used to gauge the extent to which systems are fulfilling these aspirations across the array of the World Health Organization's "building blocks" of health systems, including workforce, information systems, products and technologies, financing, leadership, governance, and stewardship.

The societal-level dignity interventions envisioned by the people we interviewed used human rights to extend dignity's upward trajectory by improving social conditions for the individuals and groups who are most marginalized. In the main, they aimed to enhance dignity by reducing asymmetry, particularly economic inequality. One woman described a plan to increase dignity by offering a government-guaranteed income:

> One of my things that I'd like to do . . . is to petition the government to give everybody a million and a half dollars. . . . For a basic million dollars you can never touch it. It's in a trust account, and you live off the interest of it every year. And the half million dollars . . . [is] just something that eases the mind. . . . Everybody gets it and you have a standard basic tax. You have opportunities open up for people who might want to start a business. . . . A lot of those serious problems would become, the things that people are putting a lot of seriousness on would become miniscule. . . . It's not going to make anybody rich, but it's going to alleviate all the worries of "can I pay my rent, can I eat."

Less imaginatively (though perhaps more feasibly), many people advocated affirmative interventions like raising the minimum wage, increasing the availability of affordable housing, legalizing drugs, making higher education free, and creating opportunity by promoting economic development in geographic and identity-based communities that traditionally have been socially excluded.

Published interventions look quite similar in their general contours. The Commission on the Social Determinants of Health (2008) endorsed three "principles of action" designed to advance health equity. Among these are to improve the material conditions of daily life, to "tackle the inequitable distribution of power, money and resources," and to raise awareness of and increase knowledge about the problem of health inequity (2). Mary Shaw, Danny Dorling, and George Davey Smith (2006) made recommendations directed at improving the material conditions of daily life by reducing social exclusion: their interventions included the passage of legislation protecting the rights of minority groups, poverty reduction through income support and progressive taxation, increased opportunities for education and employment, and targeted improvements in health system access. Similarly, Wilkinson (2005) proposed a series of policy transformations aimed at supporting what he described as social relations characterized by liberty, fraternity, and equality: greater market regulation, the promotion of government policies to equalize income distribution, more employee ownership of businesses, higher amounts of aid to the developing world, lower levels of consumption in the developed world, and education to increase public awareness of the role that social relations of inequality play in the production of poor collective health status.

The enactment of positive and negative human rights depends on a society's recognition and acceptance both of the existence of these rights and the universality of their application. Societal-level dignity interventions must actively promote such awareness and interpretation. As Anne-Emmanuelle Birn (2009) has noted in her critique of the work of the Commission on the Social Determinants of Health, many such scholarly and policy-directed discussions of how to cultivate human rights at the societal level lack explicit acknowledgment of the historical role played by political struggle in advancing collective dignity. The men and women we interviewed, particularly those who are engaged in health and human rights–related work, told me that promoting the recognition and acceptance of the rights demanded by dignity requires a multifaceted strategy encompassing both moral entrepreneurism and direct action. Such strategies are often found in dignity-focused social movements: movements of individuals and groups with shared histories of hierarchy, dispossession, and oppression who are, as Shawn Lauzon told me, "reclaiming their persons" and demanding "fairness. Equality. Access. Access to information, knowledge. Access to the knowledge of what your human right is, what you deserve as a citizen." Ultimately, these social movements aim to elevate their members' collective dignity through legal and political interventions that transform the social order. In so doing, they often make explicit their appeals to dignity.

Moral entrepreneurism seeks to draw attention to dignity violation and then to make a moral claim about it. Human rights lawyer Rebecca Cook spoke to me about the necessity of making dignity violation visible and recognizable: giving voices and faces to the victims; articulating the nature of the offense to dignity; and identifying the specific perpetrators. Failure to complete any of these steps, she noted, might lessen the impact of subsequent dignity claims. (She argued that the difficulty of identifying the perpetrators of violations characterized by omission—such as deprivation—made it more difficult to get them recognized than violations of commission—such as assault.) Similarly, street nurse Cathy Crowe described the entrepreneurial task of surfacing abnormality, or remaking as problematic that which had come to be unremarkable, like the spectacle of people sleeping (and sometimes dying) on the frigid winter streets of a wealthy city like Toronto. In effect, such dignity entrepreneurism is about raising awareness and shaping interpretation of a violation's source, locus of control, quantity, timing, execution, intention, and attribution.

Dignity-focused social movements also use direct action—like demonstrations and various forms of civil disobedience—against both the perpetrators who violate dignity and the contextual conditions that structure violation. They aim to remediate dignity violation assertively and often impolitely, not just calling attention to a violation but also intervening directly to change its qualities—seeking, for example, to make explicit the logic of a violation's malevolent attribution or to shorten the duration of a violation. In his "Letter from Birmingham

Jail" (1963), Reverend Martin Luther King Jr., who invoked human dignity as the civil rights movement's ultimate moral justification, explained how the direct action tactics adopted by the movement were necessary because they forced confrontation with race-based dignity violation: "You may well ask: 'Why direct action? Why sit-ins, marches and so forth? Isn't negotiation a better path?' You are quite right in calling for negotiation. Indeed, this is the very purpose of direct action. Nonviolent direct action seeks to create such a crisis and foster such a tension that a community which has constantly refused to negotiate is forced to confront the issue. It seeks to dramatize the issue so it can no longer be ignored." In our conversation, Ashok Bharti emphasized the need for effective social movements to address dignity violation in multiple systems:

> It's about everything that we have around us. . . . If our strategy remains limited to political systems, I guess that we can't achieve, we can't ensure dignity to everyone. Because there are economic systems that undermine the dignity of the people. There are cultural practices that undermine the dignity of the people. There are behavioral factors of the people that undermine dignity. And I don't think only the political system can address these issues. So therefore political systems, yes, but there are many more systems we need to address if we really want to push the agenda of dignity.

Several theoretical accounts exist of the forms social movements with such broad and multifaceted dignity agendas might take. In his explorations of "rankism" (hierarchy-based forms of abuse that are grounded in asymmetries of power) and its corrective, a "dignitarian movement," Fuller (2003, 2006) envisioned a society composed of institutions "in which rank-holders are held accountable, rankism is disallowed, and dignity is broadly protected" (2006, 5). The actions to be taken by a movement to promote dignity include breaking the taboos on talking about rank and its abuses, promoting recognition and awareness of rankism in many sectors of society and domains of social life, and instituting policies and practices to combat rankism and promote egalitarianism. In health care, Fuller advocated accessible services and systems designed and delivered with respect for both the users of care and the providers; in society as a whole, he called for "a more intelligent, precise, and productive sharing of authority and responsibility" (2003, 38).

Avishai Margalit (1996) conceptualized dignity as existing in opposition to humiliation, or "any sort of behavior or conditions that constitutes a sound reason for a person to consider his or her self-respect injured" (9). A social movement for dignity, then, is a social movement for "a decent society"—a society that "fights conditions which constitute a justification for its dependents to consider themselves humiliated" (10). Lindner (2006) called this kind of intervention *egalization*: "We can strive to eliminate acts of humiliation that are knowingly inflicted on others, either through individual or through institutional actions, and we can work to acquire the skills required to process feelings of humiliation without descending into mayhem and cycles of humiliation" (183). For example, although welfare societies that provide income support and other forms of social care often do so in ways that are humiliating because they institutionalize contempt, intrusion, objectification, restriction, and grouping, they can be organized in ways that minimize these dignity violations.

Rabbi Jonathan Sacks proposed a "new politics" of human dignity that attempts "to fuse a morally grounded world view . . . with a political response to the human consequences of globalisation" (Horton 2004, 1082). Sacks's book *The Dignity of Difference* (2002) highlighted the collective processes of control, contribution, compassion, creativity, cooperation, and conservation as necessary to "constructing a society of substantive justice, collective grace and equal access to the preconditions of dignity" (174). Sacks envisioned a dignity-based "global covenant . . . in which the nations of the world collectively express their commitment not only to human rights but also to human responsibilities, and not merely a political, but also an economic, environmental, moral and cultural conception of the common good, constructed on the twin foundations of shared humanity and respect for diversity" (206).

Richard Horton (2004), editor of the *Lancet*, has written that "taking account of human dignity as the over-riding requirement for a decent society might encourage us to reassess what we mean when we speak of improving global human health and advancing human development" (1085). We see dignity used in this way by the People's Health Movement (Narayan 2006), an international coalition of nongovernmental organizations dedicated to addressing the global crisis of health inequity. The preamble to the movement's founding document, the People's Charter for Health (People's Health Movement 2000), states: "Health is a social, economic and political issue and above all a fundamental human right. Inequality, poverty, exploitation, violence and injustice are at the root of ill-health and the deaths of poor and marginalized people. Health for all means that powerful interests have to be challenged, that globalization has to be opposed, and that political and economic priorities have to be drastically changed." The movement thus calls for broader recognition of the right to health and direct action against the structural challenges to this right engendered by the late capitalism, environmental degradation, and war that typify systems of hierarchy, dispossession, and oppression in a social order of inequality. It emphasizes the implementation of interventions built around strategies of grassroots organizing and greater public participation in government decision-making to promote a shift away from corporate oligarchy and toward greater democracy.

The second demand of dignity is always to acknowledge its contradictions and tensions, and thus to act and interact in ways that respect this complexity.

Bioethics, the branch of ethics in which philosophical principles are applied to moral questions in the biological sciences and the provision of health care, uses dignity in ways that highlight these contradictions and tensions, and provides a kind of cautionary tale. In intent, bioethics is both descriptive, devoted to exploring the nuances of difficult situations, and prescriptive, marshaling principle, reason, and argument to arrive at conclusions about how such difficulties might be resolved. Bioethics applies dignity both descriptively, as a factor that may be at stake in a particular situation, and prescriptively, as a principle that may provide guidance for resolving moral dilemmas.

In the broad body of bioethical work pertaining to "death with dignity," dignity appears both as an individual characteristic that is threatened by modern processes of dying in highly technological and impersonal hospital settings and as one that may be nurtured through practices that support physical and existential comfort and personal control at the end of life (Schroeder 2008; Coulehan 2007; P. R. S. Johnson 1998; Moller 1990; Sampaio 1992). In debates over physician-assisted suicide and active euthanasia, both sides invoke dignity: proponents of these practices use it in arguments that valorize autonomous choice, while opponents use it to support their arguments for the sanctity of life (Pullman 1996). It is, in part, because adversaries in such controversies are able to claim dignity that its critics malign it as "a piece of empty rhetoric full of connotation but devoid of denotation" (Birnbacher 1996, 109) and "a moral trump frayed by heavy use" (Witte 2003, 121).

Deep fault lines run throughout the landscape of the meanings and uses of dignity in bioethics. Europeans have generally embraced the concept as key to bioethical thought. It is enshrined in the German constitution (Petermann 1996), and has been cited in many court decisions and international white papers pertaining to issues in biotechnology, particularly the new tools and procedures of genetic technology (Andorno 2003; Beyleveld and Brownsword 2001; Gurnham 2005; Petermann 1996). Here, the use of dignity appears to be widely accepted, although its meanings and grounds remain a topic of some dispute and, as in the death with dignity debates, the idea is often used to argue opposite sides of a particular issue. In the United States, on the other hand, the use of dignity is itself controversial, as are its meanings and grounds, and at times all have been highly politicized. In a 2005 book review, Ashcroft summed up these fissures, describing the current conceptual status of dignity's meanings and uses among bioethicists:

> One group regards all "dignity-talk" as incoherent and at best
> unhelpful, at worst misleading. . . . Another group finds dignity talk
> illuminating in some respects, but strictly reducible to autonomy
> as extended to cover some marginal cases. . . . The third group
> considers dignity to be a concept in a family of concepts about
> capabilities, functionings, and social interactions. . . . The final
> group considers dignity as a metaphysical property possessed by all
> and only human beings, and which serves as a foundation for moral
> philosophy and human rights. (679)

Beyleveld and Brownsword (2001) produced the foundational text on the competing invocations of dignity in European biolaw and bioethics. Noting multiple examples of the ways in which dignity has been used in legal and philosophical arguments both for and against certain activities, they discerned two distinct and contradictory ways in which the concept is deployed. In the first, "dignity as empowerment," dignity is an inherent property of each human being that carries with it a set of inherent rights: "A (negative) right against unwilled interventions by others that are damaging to the circumstances or conditions that are essential if one is to flourish as a human being; and . . . a (positive) right to support and assistance in securing" such circumstances and conditions (18). In the second, "dignity as constraint," dignity inheres in "a shared vision of human dignity that reaches beyond individuals" (29). To protect this "shared vision," "those individual preferences and choices that are out of line with respect for human dignity are simply off limits" (29).

These two uses of dignity rest on different grounds. Dignity as empowerment depends on what I earlier described as the Kantian ground of capacity for moral agency, the ground based on human vulnerability, and the relational ground, all of which grant dignity to individuals. Its main uses are aspirational; it seeks to promote human flourishing and reduce human suffering. Dignity as constraint rests primarily on the metaphysical or religious ground, which is seen to confer dignity to humanity as a whole, including, through its "extended meanings" (Andorno 2003; Birnbacher 1996), to potential human beings like fetuses and future generations. Its uses are prescriptive, aimed at protecting the species against what is perceived to threaten its special status. Dignity as empowerment is invoked to support individual choice. In the physician-assisted suicide debate, it is used to argue in favor of allowing people with terminal conditions who are experiencing significant pain to determine the time and manner of their own deaths. In the same situation, dignity as constraint supports the opposite position. It is used to argue that acts of physician-assisted suicide must be forbidden because they degrade all humanity by violating the sanctity of life. Similarly, dignity as constraint would forbid the use of many biotechnologies, like cloning, holding that they threaten what is unique about being human. Dignity as empowerment, on the other hand, looks to the potential that such technologies have for alleviating misery and enhancing happiness, and thus favors their continued development.

Critics have questioned the meanings and uses of both dignity as empowerment and dignity as constraint. The fact that people with widely divergent positions on a given issue are able to claim dignity is used to deride the coherence of the concept. Because it appears to be so conceptually flexible, in practice dignity serves as simply as an emotion-based conversation stopper, an "ultimate article of faith" and thus a substitute for rational argument (Birnbacher 1996, 107). Laura Hawryluck (2004) argued that "concepts of dignity are value-laden, frequently biased" and "[without a deeper exploration of assigned meanings] risk being lost in translation" (154). Timothy Caulfield and Audrey Chapman (2005) suggested that dignity as constraint represents a knee-jerk response to elements of the new biotechnology experienced as unaesthetic or troubling—a "politically palatable articulation of the 'yuck' factor" (737). Kantian justifications for dignity as empowerment valorize autonomous moral agency, and thus are vulnerable to criticism that they leave out those who lack the circumstance or capacity for such agency (Schulman 2008; Valadier 2003). Religious justifications for dignity as constraint may be seen as incompatible with the values of pluralistic societies, in which citizens are not bound by a single theology (Becker 2001; Quante 2005). The elevation of human beings over other animals, the central tenet of human dignity, is speciesist (Beyleveld and Brownsword 2001; Birnbacher 1996). Dignity suffers from what Beyleveld and Brownsword (2001) described as the problem of "epistemological contingency"; that is, it depends on a consensual acceptance of grounds. When such a consensus is lacking, dignity loses its power (Caulfield and Chapman 2005). Thus, because the notion is so fundamentally flawed, bioethics should remain "undignified" (Cochrane 2010).

In the United States, dignity in bioethics has been a source of not just this sort of intellectual argument but also politicized controversy. In a widely cited commentary published in the *British Medical Journal* in 2003, bioethicist Ruth Macklin dismissed dignity as a "mere slogan" and "a useless concept," arguing that it had nothing of value to add to the already well-established ethical principle of respect for autonomy. It "can be eliminated," she wrote, "without any loss of content" (1420).

Her position appears to have been widely shared by many other main-stream American bioethicists, who had little conceptual use for dignity (Becker 2001; Schuklenk 2008). (By contrast, dignity's practical uses have flourished. Macklin's article occasioned a deluge of responses from clinicians, patients, and health advocates. The vast majority of these missives challenged her conclusions. "Dignity may be a useless concept to a professor of bioethics," stated one correspondent, "but it is of vital importance to clinicians and patients" [Limentani 2003]. The "eloquent, recognisable, plain language" of dignity "is instantly meaningful" in the clinic [Bastian 2003]. "I can't define dignity," wrote one doctor, "but I know it when I see it" [Rapoport 2003]. A year later, in her published reflections on a symposium examining dignity and end-of-life issues, Macklin continued to criticize dignity's conceptual fuzziness, but allowed that "dignity is not a useless concept because people use it in all sorts of ways" [2004, 212].)

However, to the members of the President's Council on Bioethics, appointed in 2002 by George W. Bush following his deliberations on the rules governing publicly funded stem cell research, dignity proved to be a highly attractive idea. Over the years of its operation, the President's Council invoked dignity in much of its work, including its published examinations of end-of-life care, cloning, and stem cells. It used dignity to argue against practices like euthanasia and to argue for restrictions on the investigation and application of new genetic technologies, but the members of the council never fully explained what they meant by dignity (Meilaender 2008). In 2008, explicitly in response to Macklin, the council produced a collection of essays intended to "take up the question of human dignity squarely, with the aim of clarifying whether and how it might be a useful concept in bioethics" (Schulman 2008, 3).

This volume, titled *Human Dignity and Bioethics* (which, not surprisingly, concluded that "dignity is anything but a useless concept" [Sulmasy 2008, 498]), became a flashpoint for criticism of the President's Council and, more broadly, for the highly restrictive version of dignity as constraint the council endorsed in its policy prescriptions. Editorializing in the journal *Bioethics*, Udo Schuklenk (2008) described the book as a defense of a "fundamentally religious notion against its secular critics" (ii), decrying the council's work as intellectually biased, politically partisan, and irrelevant to the mainstream bioethics community in the United States. Steven Pinker (2008), writing for a lay audience in the *New Republic*, pointed out the religious (mainly Catholic) nature of the authors' institutional affiliations and accused the council of providing "a moralistic justification for expanded government regulation of science, medicine, and private life" and of promoting an "obstructionist" and "theocon" bioethics. Clearly, the American controversy over dignity in bioethics was not just about bioethics; it was a microcosm of the larger cultural clash over the ideology and policies of the Bush administration.

Dignity can be vexing, and the dignity interventions I have described in this chapter may be fraught with peril. Within human dignity, the ascription of value that is justified by being human, we find tensions between exaltation and subjection, and between resistance and acceptance, as well as a number of extremely contentious arguments over what grounds this kind of dignity and how it should be applied. When put into practice, there are risks that the concept of dignity will become so politicized as to lose its usefulness. We could see societal-level dignity interventions bogged down by debates over just what constitutes "decent existence." The conditions that define decency for some may be unlivable for others. This suggests that the ways in which dignity is understood and implemented in policy must attend to social and historical context (Margalit 1996; Pullman 1996). But what has become of the universality of human dignity if we maintain these relative standards?

Social dignity is characterized by tensions between fixity and flexibility, between the ideal and the actual, between self and other, between individual and society. It is explicitly situated in time and place, but in this too the idea may be subject to conflict when implemented. Interventions that address perception, the microprocesses of awareness and interpretation—such as any future attempts to make use of the concept of "perceptual adjustment" (Matiti and Trorey 2004)—raise questions about the possible threats to dignity inherent in pathologizing people's interpretations of their own lives. The professionals who suggested to me that dignity might be promoted by helping their clients learn not to "take it personally" are well meaning, but this kind of intervention can easily be experienced as trickery. Too, by focusing on the psychology of those whose dignity is violated, such strategies may allow structurally based malignant processes and conditions of dignity violation to proliferate unexamined and unchecked.

The realities of structure and function in complex social bodies, like those of health and social care organizations and systems, mean that dignity may turn into a kind of zero-sum game. Such a consequence seems particularly likely in settings that are extremely hierarchical. The "dignity nurses" promoted by the Department of Health under the aegis of the "Dignity in Care" campaign quickly became a source of controversy (Sandler 2006). By singling out one discipline to carry the dignity banner, the intervention seemed to be denigrating the ability of other staff members to promote dignity, a slight that was interpreted by many of these personnel as a form of professional diminishment.

The zero-sum game problem becomes more acute when we turn to societal-level dignity interventions. A number of authors have noted the possibility of conflict between collective dignity and individual dignity (Bayertz 1996; Fuller 2006)—what Ignatieff (1984) termed a clash between solidarity and freedom. Despite the platitude that the dignity of all is enhanced when the dignity of one is promoted, there are also specific situations in which the dignity of the one may have to be overridden by the dignity of the many. When should we endorse dignity as empowerment and when should we endorse dignity as constraint? How do societies properly weigh and address such conflicts?

The conceptual conflicts and confusions between human and social dignity remain. Is the ground of dignity the humanity we all hold in common, or can it be found in what makes us unique? At the person level, interventions make assumptions that place them at risk of falling into a one-size-fits-all trap. That is, they may assume the particular processes and conditions of dignity violation, as well as the objects affected by violation, are the same for every individual and thus can be remedied in the same ways. But is dignity always best served by treating everyone alike? The one-size-fits-all approach is potentially paternalistic (Jacobson and Silva 2010) and in this way also impractical: when it fails, the resulting resentment is unlikely to foster greater dignity.

In organizations and systems, dignity intervention risks the one-size-fits-all conundrum on a larger scale. Specific guidelines and benchmarks may be appropriate in some contexts, but not in others, where they in fact may be harmful, either because they are ill suited to local conditions or simply poorly implemented. If nothing else, dignity must attend to nuance. Failure to do so risks facilitating violation. The advocacy organization Help the Aged has warned against the dangers of routinized approaches to dignity promotion:

> Dignity is not a formula or a recipe that can be rigidly applied from a manual. In particular, the "toolkit" approach, while useful for improving practice and as a benchmark for assessing performance, cannot fully address the "care" component of dignity in care. Indeed, a formulaic approach, taken outside the context of values and principles, can lead to a situation where all the right boxes are ticked, but still standards fall short of what older people (and other age groups) want. (Levenson 2007, 14)

The harsh circumstances that prevail in many health care service delivery organizations and systems nurture cynicism. Already, many providers told me about ways in which they use dignity instrumentally, primarily a means to an end. As dignity increasingly becomes a focus in health and social care—as it promises to do—the concept risks turning into just another category of rationalization, part of the superstructure of standardization and bureaucratization widely recognized as part of what is dehumanizing care. On the other hand, if we fail ever to specify dignity fully, it might go the route of meaninglessness, becoming nothing more than an empty slogan of rhetorical approbation, an element of the newest branding strategy.

Is dignity something inherent? Something bestowed? Something earned? The old definition of dignity as residing in a great chain of being lingers in contemporary ideas about the ways in which dignity may be conferred by achievement or renown. When notions of dignity are dependent on a parasitical domination (Draft Concept Note on Dignity 2005), or even on less malignant forms of invidious distinction, interventions that promote egalitarianism are a threat. Most of the proposed societal-level dignity interventions I have described have become the new public health orthodoxy, yet they are unsatisfying, even naïve, because they fail to engage the reality of this threat. It is easy to talk about the redistribution of political power and material wealth, but impossible to move forward without an analysis that accounts for those actors who will be threatened by these transformations, and how far they will go to resist them—resistance that is, from their perspectives, a kind of defensive dignity work. (The pushback against epidemiological studies of the impact of social inequality on the health of populations provides one illustration of this resistance [Saunders 2010]. Common respect—the dignity of one as necessary for the dignity of all—shows itself vulnerable to epistemological contingency.)

Dignity's second demand may be answered, at least in part, through more careful consideration, planning, and evaluation. The men and women we interviewed often mused about the possibility of conducing "dignity audits" or "dignity screens"—either informally, such as when making personal decisions about divergent courses of action or, more formally, to assess organizations or systems. This notion has been explored by Fuller (2006), who wrote about "dignity impact studies" in which one would build "a model of each proposed use of power in advance so as to predict its ripple effects" (34) and by Seltser and Miller (1993), who suggested using "dignity impact statements" as a way of applying "human dignity criteria . . . to social policies": "For example, our legislators should ask what are the effects of particular proposals and social systems upon the capacity of homeless families to regain some control over their own lives, upon their ability to see the world as predictable and dependable, and upon their ability to be treated as functioning and valuable members of American society" (118). That is, dignity may be used as a tool of assessment, a criterion against which the appropriateness of the status quo or the probable success (and possible failures) of interventions in practice or policy can be measured and judged. The model I have presented can be applied to these endeavors.

Such a procedure should be a situated analysis that takes into account all of dignity's moving parts: it should examine structure—the contextual conditions of position, relationship, setting, and social order; process—the social processes of dignity violation and dignity promotion; and outcome—the objects and consequences of dignity violation and dignity promotion. The analysis should begin with a wide-ranging exploration of dignity in a particular time and place, including an examination of which objects are being affected, the particular processes that are acting on these objects, and how local contextual conditions may be determining these processes. Used as a screen, this procedure can identify existing or potential problems with dignity in the environment. It also may serve as the first step in a dignity audit, which, in its next stage, should identify possible types (affirmative or defensive; directed at process or structure) and points (person, organizational, system, or societal-level) of dignity intervention and formulate a logic linking possible interventions and their probable effects on the objects of dignity violation and the consequences of these interventions for actors, settings, and the social order. Very importantly, at this stage the audit also should assess existing barriers to change and how these will be addressed by the intervention. The planning audit should result in a detailed scheme for implementation of the intervention.

The audit framework also can be used for formative (process) and summative (outcome) evaluation. Here, the logic linking intervention and objects should be detailed. A formative evaluation should seek to ascertain if this logic is being enacted in the intervention—that is, if the intervention strategies, as implemented, are actually addressing the identified points of intervention and are affecting the objects specified. A summative evaluation should focus on qualitative exploration and quantitative measurement of consequences to determine if the logic was sound: did the dignity intervention result in the intended effects?

The dignity screen or audit is as yet a proposal; I write of it in the conditional because I have not seen the procedure fully applied. However, in the psychiatric hospital where I used to work, I collaborated with a group that was beginning to experiment with how best to turn the model of dignity I have presented from the conceptual to the practical. This "dignity working group," composed of advanced practice clinicians (who fulfill leadership and educational roles in the hospital's clinical units) and frontline providers, including a number of peer support workers, came together after I gave a series of talks about dignity and dignity violation to hospital staff. The audiences found the talks engaging but painful. In the question and answer periods that followed, it was clear that the material I presented had touched a nerve. Indeed, I found that people's responses were evenly split between reminiscences of occasions when they or their family members had experienced violations of their dignity in health or social care settings and reflections on the ways in which they themselves, as health care providers, were implicated in the social processes and contextual conditions of dignity violation.

At meetings, members of the working group offered to one another examples of the dignity violations, both large and small, that they had experienced or witnessed at the hospital. People spoke of things like the indifference demonstrated by staff who simply stepped over patients who were collapsed in hallways or the intrusions experienced by people whose hospital-gowned bodies were displayed as they were transported from one building to another in order to receive treatment. The group analyzed these incidents in some detail, connecting them to the processes and conditions contained in the model. They discussed possible interventions that might be generally applied (my own contribution was the suggestion that upon admission all patients be issued a button reading "Ask Me About My Dignity") or that might be targeted to particularly common forms of violation thought to be easily amenable to remediation ("quick wins"). For example, a number of working group participants were sensitive to the humiliation experienced by patients who rode a hospital-owned bus for field trips and other activities. Because this bus bore on its side the hospital's name and logo, members of the working group believed passengers were stigmatized as soon as they disembarked. The suggested intervention was a form of concealment: make the bus anonymous by removing the hospital's identification from its exterior.

At this writing, unfortunately, the working group has become quiescent, a victim of the structural barriers of members' competing priorities and limited time, as well as the restrictions engendered by a recent dignity-eroding "reign of terror" at the hospital—layoffs and other bottom line–driven reorganizational practices and policies.

For a long while, I have puzzled over a statement that reads, "To be able to say what dignity is would be to describe the fundamental meaning of being human" (Meeks 1984, ix). During the years of my immersion in dignity, at some junctures these words have seemed merely grandiose and sentimental, devoid of any real significance. Yet I continue to be drawn to the quotation, and at times it has seemed to me quite profound. As I hope I have shown in my discussions of the ascriptive and descriptive aspects of dignity, dignity is too multifaceted and too complex to be reduced to a single "is" or "fundamental meaning." In its aspirational and prescriptive aspects, however—the normative program I have begun to explore in this chapter—dignity does carry one very clear message, its third demand: that we recognize dignity's moral import.

The language of dignity becomes salient *in extremis*, at times of confrontation (Ammicht-Quinn 2003). In bioethics, attention to dignity follows the challenges created by intensely experienced life events (like death) or new biotechnologies (like cloning), challenges that raise moral questions about what it means to be human. In health and human rights, dignity takes center stage when rights are threatened or violated, when individuals or populations are treated as something less than human. In health care, the conversation turns to dignity when providers or whole health care systems fail to deliver services that attend not just to the diseased person, but also to the person as human being.

Kurt Bayertz (1996) contrasted what he termed the philosophical and sociopolitical ideas of dignity, with the former "directed against 'vertical' limitations to [collective] human subjectivity," or the status of humanity vis-à-vis God and nature, and the latter aimed at "repel[ling] limitations which are threatening [to individuals] on a 'horizontal' level: limitations which originate from the actions of (other) human beings and from social circumstances and institutions created by human beings" (80). While bioethics tends to see its confrontations primarily as vertical, both health and human rights and health care perceive their major confrontations as horizontal.

Human dignity is a response to vertical challenges and thus it dominates bioethical debates. Adversaries seize on it as a principle with which to resolve difficult questions and quandaries. As I have described, however, a lack of consensus over the ground of human dignity makes its uses highly contested. Health and human rights shares a postwar history with bioethics, although those histories have diverged (Baker 2001), with, among other distinctions, bioethics tending to focus on individuals in the clinic and health and human rights on populations and public health. While human rights depend on dignity and thus on the epistemological contingency of human value, for historical reasons little energy has been devoted to arguing over the ground of human dignity. Instead, health and human rights makes almost exclusive use of social dignity as an idealistic corrective to horizontal challenges. It is social dignity, too, that is in play in the uses of dignity in health and social care. Dignity here is concrete, devoted to practical application. Because they have not been distracted by an engagement with the highly contentious issue of competing grounds for human dignity, scholars and activists in health and human rights and health care have managed to employ social dignity very fruitfully, using dignity language both to raise awareness and to shape interpretation, identifying and publicizing problems and galvanizing support for solutions.

Martin Hailer and Dietrich Ritschl (1996) questioned dignity's usefulness as a philosophical "platform" for medical ethics, but they praised its utility as a "frame-reference" that allows for the introduction of social context into ethical thinking. That is, dignity allows us to look at the ideal through the lens of the actual, and vice versa. Dignity is a morality detector, a gauge of a community or society's virtue. It is a "moral concept" that can be used "to measure the degree of decency of a civilization" (Draft Concept Note on Dignity 2005, 201), a sign that "intuitively alerts [us] to morally precarious situations long before reflective morality is able to discern the relevant details and provide the principles for a considered judgment" (Becker 2001, 61). When we sense a dignity violation in an action or interaction, we know that something is wrong.

In its balanced duality, through the processes and conditions of dignity promotion that parallel those of dignity violation, dignity also signals that which we know to be right: "Ideas about dignity are linked to beliefs about what is involved in living a good life, and to ideas of the Good more generally" (Feldman 1999, 686). As Pritchard (1972) argued, it is dignity—our own and that of others—that is the basis for our individual and collective demands for "just treatment" (310). Dignity provides us a way to recognize the good, and also with a set of practices to promote it, including what Ignatieff (1984) has described as "a shared language of the good" (14) with which we can begin to articulate our inchoate hopes and tangible plans for a better world—and for our better selves.

The "human project" of acting to remedy dignity violation and to enhance dignity promotion is also "a moral project" (Sacks 2002, 195). Dignity provides us with some guidance about how to act and to interact (and how not to act or to interact). It can help us "foster a basic moral attitude of conscientious and reasonable persons" (Becker 2001, 60), but it "is not a simple principle, plain in its meaning" (Tinder 2003, 245) that can be easily applied to answer every complex moral question. Rather, dignity directs us toward a method: toward "reflection and meditation" and "public dialogue" (ibid.) as processes that lead to the resolution of sticky moral problems. As my exploration of dignity's second demand suggests, there are no easy responses to demands for health and social care services provided with dignity or for the transformation of the social order from inequality to justice in order to promote individual and collective health. Dignity reminds us, however, that the ways in which we as a society go about responding to these demands—the judgments we make about the evidence we consider, the evidence we dismiss, the voices we listen to, those we shut out—are also moral matters.

One woman I interviewed spoke of dignity as realized only through a series of hard decisions: "You know, deciding to love someone, deciding to treat someone this way or that way. It's a lot of work and you have to wake up every day and say, OK, you know, this is who I'm going to be today, this is how I'm going to maneuver the world." Dignity demands not just that we make these decisions every day, but that we know them as moral choices.

REFERENCES

Ackerman, S. 2008. The Obama doctrine. *American Prospect*, March 24.
  prospect.org.
Ackley, B. J., and G. B. Ladwig. (Eds.) 2008. *Nursing Diagnosis Handbook: An
  Evidence-Based Guide to Planning Care*. 8th ed. St. Louis: Mosby.
Adelson, N. 2005. The embodiment of inequality: Health disparities in
  Aboriginal Canada. *Canadian Journal of Public Health 96* (Supplement 2):
  545–61.
Alexander, B. K. 2008. *The Globalisation of Addiction: A Study in Poverty of the
  Spirit*. Oxford: Oxford University Press.
Ali, K. 2005. Caste and Working Class in Pakistan. In *Defining Dignity: An
  Anthology of Dreams, Hopes and Struggles*, 75–79. New Delhi: World
  Dignity Forum and Heinrich Böll Foundation.
Ammicht-Quinn, R. 2003. Whose Dignity Is Inviolable? In *The Discourse of
  Human Dignity*, edited by R. Ammicht-Quinn, M. Junker-Kenny, and
  E. Tamez, 35–45. London: SCM Press.
Ammicht-Quinn, R., M. Junker-Kenny, and E. Tamez. 2003. Introduction: For
  Dignity. In *The Discourse of Human Dignity*, edited by R. Ammicht-Quinn,
  M. Junker-Kenny, and E. Tamez, 7–10. London: SCM Press.
Andorno, R. 2003. Human Dignity and the UNESCO Declaration on the
  Human Genome. (Discussion paper.) Cardiff, Wales: Cardiff Centre for
  Ethics, Law and Society.
Aranda, K., and A. Jones. 2010. Dignity in health-care: A critical exploration
  using feminism and theories of recognition. *Nursing Inquiry 17* (3): 248–56.
Arieli, Y. 2002. On the Necessary and Sufficient Conditions for the Emergence
  of the Doctrine of the Dignity of Man and His Rights. In *The Concept of
  Human Dignity in Human Rights Discourse*, edited by D. Kretzmer and
  E. Klein, 1–17. The Hague: Kluwer Law.
Arnason, S. 1998. Assuring dignity in means-tested entitlements programs: An
  elusive goal? *Journal of Gerontological Social Work 29* (2/3): 129–46.
Ashcroft, R. E. 2005. Making sense of dignity. *Journal of Medical Ethics 31* (11):
  679–82.
Backman, G., P. Hunt, R. Khosla, C. Jaramillo-Strauss, B. M. Fikre, C. Rumble,
  D. Pevalin, D. A. Paez, M. A. Pineda, A. Frisancho, P. Tarco, M. Motlagh,

D. Farcasanu, and C. Vladescu. 2008. Health systems and the right to health: An assessment of 194 countries. *Lancet* 372 (9655): 2047–85.

Baker, R. 2001. Bioethics and human rights: A historical perspective. *Cambridge Quarterly of Healthcare Ethics* 10 (3): 241–52.

Bales, K. 2007. *Ending Slavery: How We Free Today's Slaves.* Berkeley: University of California Press.

Barriers to ODSP: Experiences of People with Mental Health and Addictions. 2003. Toronto: Social Work Council and the Community Support and Research Unit, Centre for Addiction and Mental Health.

Bastian, H. 2003. An offensive slogan. (E-letter.) *BMJ*, December 19. bmj. journals.com.

Bates, J. 2008. Dignity is in the detail. *Nursing Standard* 22 (45): 24–25.

Bayertz, K. 1996. Human Dignity: Philosophical Origin and Scientific Erosion of an Idea. In *Sanctity of Life and Human Dignity*, edited by K. Bayertz, 73–90. Dordrecht, Netherlands: Kluwer Academic.

BBC World Service. 2009. *Outlook*, April 20.

Beach, M. C., J. Sugarman, R. L. Johnson, J. J. Arbelaz, P. S. Duggan, and L. A. Cooper. 2005. Do patients treated with dignity report higher satisfaction, adherence, and receipt of preventive care? *Annals of Family Medicine* 3 (4): 331–38.

Becker, G. K. 2001. In Search of Humanity: Human Dignity as a Basic Moral Attitude. In *The Future of Human Dignity*, edited by M. Häyry and T. Takala, 53–65. Amsterdam: Rodopi.

Ben-Ishai, E. 2012. *Fostering Autonomy: A Theory of Citizenship, the State, and Social Service Delivery.* University Park: Pennsylvania State University Press.

Betancourt, J. R., A. R. Green, R. R. King, A. Tan-McGrory, M. Cervantes, and M. Renfrew. 2009. *Improving Quality and Achieving Equity: A Guide for Hospital Leaders.* Boston: Disparities Solutions Center at Massachusetts General Hospital.

Beyleveld, D., and R. Brownsword. 2001. *Human Dignity in Bioethics and Biolaw.* Oxford: Oxford University Press.

Birn, A.-E. 2009. Making it politic(al): *Closing the Gap in a Generation;* Health equity through action on the social determinants of health. *Social Medicine* 4 (3): 166–82.

Birnbacher, D. 1996. Ambiguities in the Concept of Menschenwurde. In *Sanctity of Life and Human Dignity*, edited by K. Bayertz, 107–21. Dordrecht, Netherlands: Kluwer Academic.

Birrell, J., D. Thomas, and C. A. Jones. 2006. Promoting privacy and dignity for older patients in hospital. *Nursing Standard* 20 (18): 41–46.

Blanchard, J., and N. Lurie. 2004. R-E-S-P-E-C-T: Patient reports of disrespect in the health care setting and its impact on care. *Journal of Family Practice* 53 (9): 721–30.

Blendon, R. J., C. Schoen, C. M. DesRoches, R. Osborn, K. L. Scoles, and K. Zapert. 2002. Inequities in health care: A five-country survey. *Health Affairs* 21 (3): 182–91.

Borrell, L. N., D. R. Jacobs Jr., D. R. Williams, M. J. Pletcher, T. K. Houston, and C. I. Kiefe. 2007. Self-reported racial discrimination and substance use in the coronary artery risk development in adults study. *American Journal of Epidemiology* 166 (9): 1068–79.

Braveman, P., and S. Gruskin. 2003. Defining equity in health. *Journal of Epidemiology and Community Health* 57 (4): 254–58.

Brooker, A. S. 2008. *Dignity under Threat: Low Power and High Distress in the Service Sector.* Saarbrücken, Germany: VDM Verlag.

Butler, F. 2006. *Rights for Real: Older People, Human Rights and the CEHR.* London, UK: Age Concern Reports.

Calnan, M., D. Badcott, and G. Woolhead. 2006. Dignity under threat? A study of the experiences of older people in the United Kingdom. *International Journal of Health Services* 36 (2): 355–75.

Caulfield, T., and R. Brownsword. 2006. Human dignity: A guide to policy making in the biotechnology era? *Nature Reviews Genetics* 7 (1): 72–76.

Caulfield, T., and A. Chapman. 2005. Human dignity as a criterion for science policy. *PloS Medicine* 2 (8): 736–38.

CBC News. 2009a. Aboriginal man alleges beating, racial slurs by hospital security guards. *www.cbc.ca*, February 12.

CBC News. 2009b. Nurse alleges previous incident of beating by St. Mike's security. *www.cbc.ca*, February 13.

CBC News. 2009c. Beatings of homeless people not unusual: Former hospital security guard. *www.cbc.ca*, February 18.

Centre for Research on Inner City Health. 2009. *Measuring Equity of Care in Hospital Settings: From Concepts to Indicators.* Toronto: St. Michael's Hospital.

Chan, C. K., and G. Bowpitt. 2005. *Human Dignity and Welfare Systems.* Bristol, UK: Policy Press.

Chapman, A. R. 2009. Globalization, human rights, and the social determinants of health. *Bioethics* 23 (2): 97–111.

Chilton, M. 2006. Developing a measure of dignity for stress-related health outcomes. *Health and Human Rights* 9 (2): 208–33.

Chochinov, H. M. 2002. Dignity-conserving care—a new model for palliative care. *JAMA* 287 (17): 2253–60.

Chochinov, H. M. 2003. Defending dignity. *Palliative and Supportive Care* 1 (4): 307–8.

Chochinov, H. M. 2004. Dignity and the eye of the beholder. *Journal of Clinical Oncology* 22 (7): 1336–40.

Chochinov, H. M. 2007. Dignity and the essence of medicine: The A, B, C, and D of dignity conserving care. *BMJ* 335 (7612): 184–87.

Chochinov, H. M., T. Hack, S. McClement, L. Kristjanson, and M. Harlos. 2002. Dignity in the terminally ill: A developing empirical model. *Social Science and Medicine* 54 (3): 433–43.

Christakis, N. 2007. The Social Origins of Dignity in Medical Care at the End of Life. In *Perspectives on Human Dignity: A Conversation*, edited by J. Malpas and N. Lickis, 199–207. Dordrecht, Netherlands: Springer.

Cochrane, A. 2010. Undignified bioethics. *Bioethics* 24 (5): 234–41.

Commission on the Social Determinants of Health. 2008. *Closing the Gap in a Generation: Health Equity through Action on the Social Determinants of Health; Final Report of the Commission on Social Determinants of Health.* Geneva: World Health Organization.

Committee on Economic, Social and Cultural Rights. 2000. General Comment 14: The Right to the Highest Attainable Standard of Health (Article 12 of the International Covenant on Economic, Social and Cultural Rights). In *Health and Human Rights: Basic International Documents*, edited by S. P. Marks. Boston: François-Xavier Bagnoud Center for Health and Human Rights.

Cooley, C. H. [1902] 1983. *Human Nature and the Social Order.* New Brunswick, NJ: Transaction Books.

Copp, L. A. 1997. Stealing a nurse's human dignity. *Journal of Professional Nursing* 13 (2): 63–64.

Coulehan, J. 2007. Dying with Dignity: The Story Reveals Its Meaning. In *Perspectives on Human Dignity: A Conversation*, edited by J. Malpas and N. Lickis, 209–23. Dordrecht, Netherlands: Springer.

Courtwright, A. M. 2009. Justice, stigma, and the new epidemiology of health disparities. *Bioethics* 23 (2): 90–96.

Coventry, M. L. 2006. Care with dignity: A concept analysis. *Journal of Gerontological Nursing* 32 (5): 42–48.

Dales, R. C. 1977. A medieval view of human dignity. *Journal of the History of Ideas* 38 (4): 557–72.

Danner, M. 2009. U.S. torture: Voices from the black sites. *New York Review of Books*, April 9.

Das, B. 2005. The Virtue of Being Human—Right to Dignity. Translated by Pamposh Kumar. In *Defining Dignity: An Anthology of Dreams, Hopes and Struggles*, 132–45. New Delhi: World Dignity Forum and Heinrich Böll Foundation.

De Vogli, R., J. E. Ferrie, T. Chandola, M. Kivimake, and M. G. Marmot. 2007. Unfairness and health: Evidence from the Whitehall Study. *Journal of Epidemiology and Community Health* 61 (6): 513–18.

Dicke, K. 2002. The Founding Function of Human Dignity in the Universal Declaration of Human Rights. In *The Concept of Human Dignity in Human Rights Discourse*, edited by D. Kretzmer and E. Klein, 111–20. The Hague: Kluwer Law.

Dillon, R. S. 1995. Introduction. In *Dignity, Character, and Self-Respect*, edited by R. S. Dillon, 1–49. New York: Routledge.

Discrimination and Health. 2006. *A Threat to Public Health: Final Report of the Health and Discrimination Project.* Sweden: National Institute of Public Health.

Draft Concept Note on Dignity. 2005. In *Defining Dignity: An Anthology of*

Dreams, Hopes and Struggles, 200–204. New Delhi: World Dignity Forum and Heinrich Böll Foundation.

Dussel, E. 2003. Dignity: Its Denial and Recognition in a Specific Context of Liberation. In *The Discourse of Human Dignity*, edited by R. Ammicht-Quinn, M. Junker-Kenny, and E. Tamez, 93–104. London: SCM Press.

Edel, A. 1969. Humanist Ethics and the Meaning of Human Dignity. In *Moral Problems in Contemporary Society*, edited by P. Kurtz, 227–40. Englewood Cliffs, NJ: Prentice-Hall.

Educating for Dignity: A Multidisciplinary Workbook. [c. 2004.] Cardiff: Dignity and Older Europeans. Available at *medic.cardiff.ac.uk*.

Ehrenreich, B. 2001. *Nickel and Dimed: On (Not) Getting by in America*. New York: Metropolitan Books.

Equality and Human Rights Group. 2008. *Human Rights in Healthcare—A Framework for Local Action*. London: Skipton House.

Fanon, F. 1963. *The Wretched of the Earth*. Translated by C. Farrington. New York: Grove Press.

Farmer, P. 2005. *Pathologies of Power*. Berkeley: University of California Press.

Feder-Alford, E. 2006. Only a piece of meat: One patient's reflections on her eight-day hospital experience. *Qualitative Inquiry* 12 (3): 596–620.

Feinberg, J. 1970. The nature and value of rights. *Journal of Value Inquiry* 4 (4): 243–60.

Feldman, D. 1999. Human dignity as a legal value—Part I. *Public Law*, Winter 1999: 682–702.

Feldman, D. 2000. Human dignity as a legal value—Part II. *Public Law*, Spring 2000: 61–76.

Fischlin, D., and M. Nandorfy. 2007. *The Concise Guide to Global Human Rights*. Montreal: Black Rose Books.

Fisher, M. F. K. 1997. *A Life in Letters: Correspondence, 1929–1991*. Washington, DC: Counterpoint.

Franklin, L.-L., B.-M. Ternestedt, and L. Nordenfelt. 2006. Views on the dignity of elderly nursing home residents. *Nursing Ethics* 13 (2): 130–46.

Fuller, R. W. 2003. *Somebodies and Nobodies: Overcoming the Abuse of Rank*. Gabriola Island, Canada: New Society.

Fuller, R. W. 2006. *All Rise: Somebodies, Nobodies, and the Politics of Dignity*. San Francisco: Berrett-Koehler.

Gallagher, A., S. Li, P. Wainwright, I. R. Jones, and D. Lee. 2008. Dignity in the care of older people—a review of the theoretical and empirical literature. *BMC Nursing* 7 (11). *www.biomedcentral.com*.

Gardner, B. 2008. *Health Equity Discussion Paper*. Toronto: Toronto Central LHIN.

Gaylin, W. 1984. In defense of the dignity of being human. *Hastings Center Report*, August 1984: 18–22.

George, L. K. 1998. Dignity and the quality of life in old age. *Journal of Gerontological Social Work* 29 (2/3): 39–52.

Gewirth, A. 1992. Human Dignity as the Basis of Rights. In *The Constitution of Rights: Human Dignity and American Values,* edited by M. J. Meyer and W. A. Parent, 10–28. Ithaca, NY: Cornell University Press.

Goffman, E. 1961. *Asylums.* New York: Anchor.

Goffman, E. 1963. *Stigma: Notes on the Management of Spoiled Identity.* Englewood Cliffs, NJ: Prentice-Hall.

Goodin, R. E. 1981. The political theories of choice and dignity. *American Philosophical Quarterly* 18 (2): 91–100.

Griffin-Heslin, V. L. 2005. An analysis of the concept dignity. *Accident and Emergency Nursing* 13 (4): 251–57.

Gruskin, S., and D. Tarantola. 2000. Health and Human Rights. François-Xavier Bagnoud Center for Health and Human Rights Working Paper Series, No.10. Boston: Harvard School of Public Health.

Gurnham, D. 2005. The mysteries of human dignity and the brave new world of human cloning. *Social and Legal Studies* 14 (2): 197–214.

Guru, G. 2005. Dignity and New Morality. (Gopal Guru speaks to Ramesh Upadhhyana.) Translated by Nandini Chandra. In *Defining Dignity: An Anthology of Dreams, Hopes and Struggles,* 31–47. New Delhi: World Dignity Forum and Heinrich Böll Foundation.

Hailer, M., and D. Ritschl. 1996. The General Notion of Human Dignity and the Specific Arguments in Medical Ethics. In *Sanctity of Life and Human Dignity,* edited by K. Bayertz, 91–106. Dordrecht, Netherlands: Kluwer Academic.

Hall, P. A., and M. Lamont. (Eds.) 2009. *Successful Societies: How Institutions and Culture Affect Health.* New York: Cambridge University Press.

Harris, G. W. 1997. *Dignity and Vulnerability.* Berkeley: University of California Press.

Hawryluck, L. 2004. Lost in translation: Dignity dialogues at the end of life. *Journal of Palliative Care* 20 (3): 150–54.

Häyry, M. 2004. Another look at dignity. *Cambridge Quarterly of Healthcare Ethics* 13 (1): 7–14.

Healthcare Commission. 2007. *Caring for Dignity: A National Report on Dignity in Care for Older People While in Hospital.* London: Commission for Healthcare Audit and Inspection.

Hill, T. E. 1992. *Dignity and Practical Reason in Kant's Moral Theory.* Ithaca, NY: Cornell University Press.

Hodson, R. 2001. *Dignity at Work.* Cambridge: Cambridge University Press.

Hoffman, L., and B. Coffey. 2008. Dignity and indignation: How people experiencing homelessness view services and providers. *Social Science Journal* 45 (2): 207–22.

Honneth, A. 1995. *The Struggle for Recognition: The Moral Grammar of Social Conflicts.* Translated by J. Anderson. Cambridge: Polity Press.

Hooks, G., and C. Mosher. 2005. Outrages against personal dignity: Rationalizing abuse and torture in the war on terror. *Social Forces* 83 (4): 1627–46.

Horton, R. 2004. Rediscovering human dignity. *Lancet* 364 (9439): 1081–85.

Hughes, A., B. Davies, and M. Gudmundsdottir. 2008. "Can you give me respect?": Experiences of the urban poor on a dedicated AIDS nursing home unit. *Journal of the Association of Nurses in AIDS Care* 19 (5): 343–56.

Iezzoni, L. 1999. Boundaries. *Health Affairs* 18 (6): 171–76.

Ignatieff, M. 1984. *The Needs of Strangers*. London: Chatto and Windus.

Ignatieff, M. 2001. *Human Rights as Politics and Idolatry*. Princeton, NJ: Princeton University Press.

Ignatius, D. 2007. The dignity agenda. *Washington Post*, October 14.

International Committee of the Red Cross. 2007. ICRC Report on the Treatment of Fourteen "High Value Detainees" in CIA Custody. *www.nybooks.com/media/doc/2010/04/22/icrc-report.pdf*.

International Covenant on Civil and Political Rights. 1966. Adopted and opened for signature, ratification, and accession by United Nations General Assembly Resolution 2200 A (XXI) on December 16, 1966. Entered into force on March 23, 1976, in accordance with Article 49. *www.un.org/millennium/law/iv-4.htm*.

International Covenant on Economic, Social, and Cultural Rights. 1966. Adopted and opened for signature, ratification, and accession by United Nations General Assembly Resolution 2200 A (XXI) on December 16, 1966. Entered into force on January 3, 1976, in accordance with Article 49. *treaties.un.org*.

Ishiguro, K. 1989. *The Remains of the Day*. London: Faber and Faber.

Jacelon, C. S. 2003. The dignity of elders in an acute care hospital. *Qualitative Health Research* 13 (4): 543–56.

Jacelon, C. S., T. W. Connelly, R. Brown, K. Proulx, and T. Vo. 2004. A concept analysis of dignity for older adults. *Journal of Advanced Nursing* 48 (1): 76–83.

Jackson, M., and G. Stewart. 2009. A Flawed Compass: A Human Rights Analysis of the Roadmap to Strengthening Public Safety. Available at *ssrn.com/abstract=1881036*.

Jacobs, B. B. 2000. Respect for human dignity in nursing: Philosophical and practical perspectives. *Canadian Journal of Nursing Research* 32 (2): 15–33.

Jacobs, B. B. 2001. Respect for human dignity: A central phenomenon to philosophically unit nursing theory and practice through consilience of knowledge. *Advances in Nursing Science* 24 (1): 17–35.

Jacobson, N. 2007. Dignity and health: A review. *Social Science and Medicine* 64 (2): 292–302.

Jacobson, N. 2009a. A taxonomy of dignity: A grounded theory study. *BMC International Health and Human Rights* 9 (3). *www.biomedcentral.com*.

Jacobson, N. 2009b. Dignity violation in health care. *Qualitative Health Research* 19 (11): 1536–47.

Jacobson, N., and C. S. Dewa. 2009. *The Peer Program at the Centre for Addiction and Mental Health: A Participatory Evaluation*. Toronto: Centre for Addiction and Mental Health.

Jacobson, N., and D. Silva. 2010. Dignity promotion and beneficence. *Journal of Bioethical Inquiry* 7 (4): 365–72.

Jacobson, N., V. Oliver, and A. Koch. 2009. An urban geography of dignity. *Health and Place* 15 (3): 695–701.

James, P. D. 1992. *The Children of Men*. Toronto: Knopf.

Johnson, J. P. 1971. Human dignity and the nature of society. In *Human Dignity: This Century and the Next*, edited by R. Gotesky and E. Laszlo, 317–52. New York: Gordon and Breach.

Johnson, P. R. S. 1998. An analysis of "dignity." *Theoretical Medicine and Bioethics* 19 (4): 337–52.

Johnston, V., P. Allotey, K. Mulholland, and M. Markovic. 2009. Measuring the health impact of human rights violations related to Australian asylum policies and practices: A mixed methods study. *BMC International Health and Human Rights* 9 (1). *www.biomedcentral.com*.

Jones, A., and K. Aranda. 2009. Putting dignity first. *Community Practitioner* 82 (8): 30–32.

Karcher, S. 2001. In My Fingertips I Don't Have a Soul Anymore. In *At the Side of Torture Survivors*, edited by S. Graessner, N. Gurris, and C. Pross, and translated by J. M. Riemer, 70–94. Baltimore: Johns Hopkins University Press.

Kawachi, I., N. E. Adler, and W. H. Dow. 2010. Money, schooling, and health: Mechanisms and causal evidence. *Annals of the New York Academy of Sciences* 1186 (1): 56–58.

Khandor, E., and K. Mason. 2007. *The Street Health Report*. Toronto: Streethealth.

Kilbourne, A. M., G. Switzer, K. Hyman, M. Crowley-Matoka, and M. J. Fine. 2006. Advancing health disparities research within the health care system: A conceptual framework. *American Journal of Public Health* 96 (12): 2113–21.

Killmister, S. 2010. Dignity: Not such a useless concept. *Journal of Medical Ethics* 36 (3): 160–64.

King, M. L., Jr. 1963. Letter from Birmingham Jail. Available at the Martin Luther King, Jr., Research and Education Institute website, *mlk-kpp01.stanford.edu*.

Kittay, E. 2003. Disability, Equal Dignity and Care. In *The Discourse of Human Dignity*, edited by R. Ammicht-Quinn, M. Junker-Kenny, and E. Tamez, 105–15. London: SCM Press.

Klein, E. 2002. Human Dignity in German law. In *The Concept of Human Dignity in Human Rights Discourse*, edited by D. Kretzmer and E. Klein, 145–59. The Hague: Kluwer Law.

Knowles, L. P. 2001. The lingua franca of human rights and the rise of a global bioethic. *Cambridge Quarterly of Healthcare Ethics* 10 (3): 253–63.

Kolnai, A. 1995. Dignity. In *Dignity, Character, and Self-Respect*, edited by R. S. Dillon, 53–75. New York: Routledge.

Kondo, N., G. Sembajwe, I. Kawachi, R. M. van Dam, S. V. Subramanian, and

Z. Yamagata. 2009. Income inequality, mortality, and self rated health: Meta-analysis of multilevel studies. *BMJ* 339 (November 10). *www.bmj.com.*

Kraynak, R. P. 2003. "Made in the Image of God": The Christian View of Human Dignity and Political Order. In *In Defense of Human Dignity: Essays for Our Times*, edited by R. P. Kraynak and G. Tinder, 81–118. Notre Dame, IN: University of Notre Dame Press.

Krieger, N. 2001. Theories for social epidemiology in the 21st century: An ecosocial perspective. *International Journal of Epidemiology* 30 (4): 668–77.

Krieger, N. 2005. Embodiment: A conceptual glossary for epidemiology. *Journal of Epidemiology and Community Health* 59 (5): 350–55.

Lawrence-Lightfoot, S. 1999. *Respect.* Reading, MA: Perseus.

Levenson, R. 2007. *The Challenge of Dignity in Care.* London: Help the Aged.

Levi, P. 1959. *Survival in Auschwitz: If This Is a Man.* Translated by S. Woolf. New York: Orion Press.

Levi, P. 1989. *The Drowned and the Saved.* Translated by R. Rosenthal. New York: Vintage.

Liebenberg, S. 2005. The value of human dignity in interpreting socio-economic rights. *South African Journal on Human Rights* 21 (2): 1–31.

Limentani, A. E. 2003. Scientific moral imperialism. (E-letter.) *BMJ*, December 23. bmj.journals.com.

Lindner, E. 2006. *Making Enemies: Humiliation and International Conflict.* Westport, CT: Praeger Security.

Lothian, K., and I. Philp. 2001. Maintaining the dignity and autonomy of older people in the healthcare setting. *BMJ* 322 (7287): 668–70.

Luban, D. 2009. Human dignity, humiliation, and torture. *Kennedy Institute of Ethics Journal* 19 (3): 211–30.

Lundqvist, A., and T. Nilstun. 2007. Human dignity in paediatrics: The effects of health care. *Nursing Ethics* 14 (2): 215–28.

Lynch, G. W. (Ed.) 1999. *Human Dignity and the Police: Ethics and Integrity in Police Work.* Springfield, IL: Charles C. Thomas.

Lynch, J., G. D. Smith, S. Harper, M. Hillemeier, N. Ross, G. A. Kaplan, and M. Wolfson. 2004. Is income inequality a determinant of population health? Part I. A systematic review. *Milbank Quarterly* 82 (1): 5–99.

Lynd, H. M. 1958. *On Shame and the Search for Identity.* New York: Wiley.

Macklin, R. 2003. Dignity is a useless concept. *BMJ* 327 (7429): 1419–20.

Macklin, R. 2004. Reflections on the human dignity symposium: Is dignity a useless concept? *Journal of Palliative Care* 20 (3): 212–16.

Magee, H., S. Parsons, and J. Askham. 2008. *Measuring Dignity in Care for Older People.* Oxford: Picker Institute Europe.

Mairis, E. D. 1994. Concept clarification in professional practice—dignity. *Journal of Advanced Nursing* 19 (5): 947–53.

Malpas, J. 2007. Human Dignity and Human Being. In *Perspectives on Human Dignity: A Conversation*, edited by J. Malpas and N. Lickis, 19–25. Dordrecht, Netherlands: Springer.

Malterud, K., and J. Thesen. 2008. When the helper humiliates the patient: A qualitative study about unintended humiliations. *Scandinavian Journal of Public Health* 36 (1): 92–98.

Mangset, M., T. E. Dahl, R. Forde, and T. B. Wyller. 2008. "We're just sick people, nothing else": . . . Factors contributing to elderly stroke patients' satisfaction with rehabilitation. *Clinical Rehabilitation* 22 (9): 825–35.

Mann, J. M. 1997. Medicine and public health, ethics and human rights. *Hastings Center Report* 27 (3): 6–13.

Mann, J. M. 1998. Dignity and health: The UDHR's revolutionary first article. *Health and Human Rights* 3 (2): 31–38.

Mann, J. M., L. Gostin, S. Gruskin, T. Brennan, Z. Lazzarini, and H. Fineberg. 1999. Health and Human Rights. In *Health and Human Rights: A Reader*, edited by J. M. Mann, S. Gruskin, M. A. Grodin, and G. J. Annas, 7–20. New York: Routledge.

Marcel, G. 1963. *The Existential Background of Human Dignity*. Cambridge, MA: Harvard University Press.

Margalit, A. 1996. *The Decent Society*. Translated by N. Goldblum. Cambridge, MA: Harvard University Press.

Marks, S. P. 2003. Health from a Human Rights Perspective. François-Xavier Bagnoud Center for Health and Human Rights Working Paper Series, No. 14. Boston: Harvard School of Public Health.

Marmot, M. 2004. Dignity and inequality. *Lancet* 364 (9439): 1019–21.

Marmot, M., and R. G. Wilkinson. (Eds.) 2006. *Social Determinants of Health*. 2nd ed. Oxford: Oxford University Press.

Matiti, M. R., E. Cotrel-Gibbons, and K. Teasdale. 2007. Promoting patient dignity in healthcare settings. *Nursing Standard* 21 (45): 46–52.

Matiti, M. R., and G. M. Trorey. 2004. Perceptual adjustment levels: Patients' perception of their dignity in the hospital setting. *International Journal of Nursing Studies* 41 (7): 735–44.

Matiti, M. R., and G. M. Trorey. 2008. Patients' expectations of the maintenance of their dignity. *Journal of Clinical Nursing* 17 (20): 2709–17.

Matthews, K. A., L. C. Gallo, and S. E. Taylor. 2010. Are psychosocial factors mediators of socioeconomic status and health connections? *Annals of the New York Academy of Sciences* 1186 (February): 146–73.

Mayer, J. 2005. The experiment. *New Yorker*, July 10.

Mays, V. M., S. D. Cochran, and N. W. Barnes. 2007. Race, race-based discrimination, and health outcomes among African Americans. *Annual Review of Psychology* 58 (January): 201–25.

McDougal, M. S., H. Lasswell, and L. Chen. 1980. *Human Rights and the World Public Order: The Basic Policies of an International Law of Human Dignity*. New Haven, CT: Yale University Press.

McEwen, B. S., and P. J. Gianaros. 2010. Central role of the brain in stress and adaptation: Links to socioeconomic status, health, and disease. *Annals of the New York Academy of Sciences* 1186 (February): 190–222.

Mead, G. H. [1934] 1962. The Self, the I, and the Me. In *Mind, Self, and Society:*

From the Standpoint of a Social Behaviorist, edited by C. W. Morris, 136–44, 195–96. Chicago: University of Chicago Press.

Mead, L. M. 1997. The Rise of Paternalism. In *The New Paternalism: Supervisory Approaches to Poverty*, edited by L. M. Mead, 1–38. Washington, DC: Brookings Institution Press.

Meeks, M. D. 1984. Introduction. In *On Human Dignity: Political Theory and Ethics*, J. Moltmann, translated by M. D. Meeks, ix–xiv. Philadelphia: Fortress Press.

Meilaender, G. 2008. Human Dignity: The Council's Vision. In *Human Dignity and Bioethics: Essays Commissioned by the President's Council on Bioethics*, 253–77. Washington, DC: President's Council on Bioethics.

Meyer, M. J. 1989. Dignity, rights, and self-control. *Ethics 99* (3): 520–34.

Meyer, M. J. 2002. Dignity as a (Modern) Virtue. In *The Concept of Human Dignity in Human Rights Discourse*, edited by D. Kretzmer and E. Klein, 195–207. The Hague: Kluwer Law.

Miller, A. B., and C. B. Keys. 2001. Understanding dignity in the lives of homeless persons. *American Journal of Community Psychology 29* (2): 331–54.

Milton, C. L. 2008. The ethics of human dignity: A nursing theoretical perspective. *Nursing Science Quarterly 21* (3): 207–10.

Moller, D. W. 1990. *On Death without Dignity: The Human Impact of Technological Dying*. New York: Baywood.

Moody, H. 1998. Why dignity in old age matters. *Journal of Gerontological Social Work 29* (2/3): 13–38.

Morsink, J. 1999. *The Universal Declaration of Human Rights: Origins, Drafting, and Intent*. Philadelphia: University of Pennsylvania Press.

Narayan, R. 2006. The role of the People's Health Movement in putting the social determinants of health on the global agenda. *Health Promotion Journal of Australia 17* (3): 186–88.

Nazroo, J. Y., and D. R. Williams. 2006. The Social Determination of Ethnic/ Racial Inequalities in Health. In *Social Determinants of Health*, 2nd ed., edited by M. Marmot and R. G. Wilkinson, 238–66. Oxford: Oxford University Press.

Nordenfelt, L. 2003. Dignity and the care of the elderly. *Medicine, Health Care and Philosophy 6* (2): 103–10.

Nordenfelt, L. 2004. The varieties of dignity. *Health Care Analysis 12* (2): 69–81.

Nussbaum, M. C. 2000. *Women and Human Development: The Capabilities Approach*. Cambridge: Cambridge University Press.

O'Mathuna, D. P. 2006. Human dignity in the Nazi era: Implications for contemporary bioethics. *BMC Medical Ethics 7* (2). *www.biomedcentral.com.*

Oyaya, C. O., and D. C. O. Kaseje. 2001. Health, poverty and dignified living. *Development 44* (1): 51–57.

Paradies, Y. 2006. A systematic review of empirical research on self-reported racism and health. *International Journal of Epidemiology 35* (4): 888–901.

Parsons, A., and C. Hooker. 2010. Dignity and narrative medicine. *Journal of Bioethical Inquiry 7* (4): 345–51.

Paust, J. J. 1984. Human dignity as a constitutional right: A jurisprudentially based inquiry into criteria and content. *Howard Law Journal* 27 (1): 145–225.

People's Health Movement. 2000. People's Charter for Health. In *Health and Human Rights: Basic International Documents*, edited by S. P. Marks. Boston: François-Xavier Bagnoud Center for Health and Human Rights.

Petermann, T. 1996. Human Dignity and Genetic Tests. In *Sanctity of Life and Human Dignity*, edited by K. Bayertz, 123–38. Dordrecht, Netherlands: Kluwer Academic.

Pico della Mirandola, G. [1468] 1948. Oration on the Dignity of Man. In *The Renaissance Philosophy of Man*, edited by E. Cassirer, P. O. Kristeller, and J. H. Randall Jr., 223–54. Chicago: University of Chicago Press.

Pinker, S. 2008. The stupidity of dignity. *New Republic*, May 28.

Pleschberger, S. 2007. Dignity and the challenge of dying in nursing homes: The residents' view. *Age and Aging* 36 (2): 197–202.

Powers, M., and R. Faden. 2006. *Social Justice: The Moral Foundations of Public Health and Health Policy*. New York: Oxford University Press.

Pritchard, M. S. 1972. Human dignity and justice. *Ethics* 82 (4): 299–313.

Pullman, D. 1996. Dying with dignity and the death of dignity. *Health Law Journal* 4: 197–219.

Pullman, D. 1999. The ethics of autonomy and dignity in long-term care. *Canadian Journal on Aging* 18 (1): 26–46.

Pullman, D. 2002. Human dignity and the ethics and aesthetics of pain and suffering. *Theoretical Medicine* 23 (1): 75–94.

Quante, M. 2005. Quality of life assessment and human dignity: Against the incompatibility-assumption. *Poiesis and Praxis* 3 (3): 168–80.

Raphael, D. (Ed.) 2004. *Social Determinants of Health: Canadian Perspectives*. Toronto: Canadian Scholars' Press.

Rapoport, J. 2003. Dignity a useless concept?? (E-letter.) *BMJ*, December 22. bmj.journals.com.

Rayman, P. M. 2001. *Beyond the Bottom Line: The Search for Dignity at Work*. New York: Palgrave.

Reutter, L. I., M. J. Stewart, G. Veenstra, R. Love, D. Raphael, and E. Makwarimba. 2009. "Who do they think we are, anyway?": Perceptions of and responses to poverty stigma. *Qualitative Health Research* 19 (3): 297–311.

Ritschl, D. 2008. Ethical Maxims from Theological Concepts of Human Dignity? In *The Concept of Human Dignity in Human Rights Discourse*, edited by D. Kretzmer and E. Klein, 87–98. The Hague: Kluwer Law.

Rosen, G. [1958] 1993. *A History of Public Health*. Expanded edition. Baltimore: Johns Hopkins University Press.

Sacks, J. 2002. *The Dignity of Difference*. London: Continuum.

Sampaio, L. 1992. To die with dignity. *Social Science and Medicine* 35 (4): 433–41.

Sandler, C. 2006. Standing up for dignity. *Nursing Standard* 21 (8): 20–22.

Saunders, P. 2010. *Beware False Prophets: Equality, the Good Society, and "The Spirit Level."* London: Policy Exchange.

Schachter, O. 1983. Human dignity as a normative concept. *American Journal of International Law* 77 (4): 848–54.

Scheff, T. J. 1994. *Bloody Revenge: Emotions, Nationalism, and War.* Boulder, CO: Westview Press.

Scheff, T. J., S. M. Retzinger, and M. T. Ryan. 1989. Crime, Violence, and Self-Esteem: Review and Proposals. In *The Social Importance of Self-Esteem,* edited by A. M. Mecca, N. J. Smelser, and J. Vasconcellos, 165–94. Berkeley: University of California Press.

Schlink, B. 1998. *The Reader.* New York: Vintage.

Schroeder, D. 2008. Dignity: Two riddles and four concepts. *Cambridge Quarterly of Healthcare Ethics* 17 (2): 230–38.

Schüklenk, U. 2008. National bioethics commissions and partisan politics. (Editorial.) *Bioethics* 22 (6): ii–iii.

Schulman, A. 2008. Bioethics and the Question of Human Dignity. In *Human Dignity and Bioethics: Essays Commissioned by the President's Council on Bioethics,* 3–17. Washington, DC: President's Council on Bioethics.

Seabrook, J. 2005. Dignity and Its Paradoxes. In *Defining Dignity: An Anthology of Dreams, Hopes and Struggles,* 146–51. New Delhi: World Dignity Forum and Heinrich Böll Foundation.

Seeman, T. E., B. S. McEwen, J. W. Rowe, and B. H. Singer. 2001. Allostatic load as a marker of cumulative biological risk: MacArthur studies of successful aging. *PNAS* 98 (8): 4770–75.

Seeman, T., E. Epel, T. Gruenewald, A. Karlamangla, and B. S. McEwen. 2010. Socio-economic differentials in peripheral biology: Cumulative allostatic load. *Annals of the New York Academy of Sciences* 1186 (February): 223–39.

Seltser, B. J., and D. E. Miller. 1993. *Homeless Families: The Struggle for Dignity.* Urbana: University of Illinois Press.

Sen, A. 1999. *Commodities and Capabilities.* New Delhi: Oxford University Press.

Sennett, R. 2003. *Respect in a World of Inequality.* New York: Norton.

Sennett, R., and J. Cobb. 1972. *The Hidden Injuries of Class.* New York: Vintage.

Sharma, M., and A. Bharti. 2005. In Lieu of an Introduction. In *Defining Dignity: An Anthology of Dreams, Hopes and Struggles,* 2–12. New Delhi: World Dignity Forum and Heinrich Böll Foundation.

Shaw, M., D. Dorling, and G. D. Smith. 2006. Poverty, Social Exclusion, and Minorities: The Social Determination of Ethnic/Racial Inequalities in Health. In *Social Determinants of Health,* 2nd ed., edited by M. Marmot and R. G. Wilkinson, 196–223. Oxford: Oxford University Press.

Shell, S. M. 2003. Kant on Human Dignity. In *In Defense of Human Dignity: Essays for Our Times,* edited by R. P. Kraynak and G. Tinder, 53–80. Notre Dame, IN: University of Notre Dame Press.

Shotton, L., and D. Seedhouse. 1998. Practical dignity in caring. *Nursing Ethics* 5 (3): 246–55.

Silver, M., R. Conte, M. Miceli, and I. Poggi. 1986. Humiliation: Feeling, social control and the construction of identity. *Journal for the Theory of Social Behaviour* 16 (3): 269–83.

Simpson, E. 2004. Harms to dignity, bioethics, and the scope of biolaw. *Journal of Palliative Care* 20 (3): 185–92.

Smelser, N. J. 1989. Self-Esteem and Social Problems: An Introduction. In *The Social Importance of Self-Esteem*, edited by A. M. Mecca, N. J. Smelser, and J. Vasconcellos, 1–25. Berkeley: University of California Press.

Snow, D. A., and L. Anderson. 1987. Identity work among the homeless: The verbal construction and avowal of personal identities. *American Journal of Sociology* 92 (6): 1336–71.

Soderberg, S., B. Lundman, and A. Norberg. 1999. Struggling for dignity: The meaning of women's experiences of living with fibromyalgia. *Qualitative Health Research* 9 (5): 575–87.

Soderberg, A., F. Gilje, and A. Norberg, 1997. Dignity in situations of ethical difficulty in intensive care. *Intensive and Critical Care Nursing* 13 (3): 135-44.

Spiegelberg, H. 1970. Human Dignity: A Challenge to Contemporary Philosophy. In *Human Dignity: This Century and the Next*, edited by R. Gotesky and E. Laszlo, 39–64. New York: Gordon and Breach.

Stabell, A., and D. Naden. 2006. Patients' dignity in a rehabilitation ward: Ethical challenges for nursing staff. *Nursing Ethics* 13 (3): 236–48.

Statman, D. 2000. Humiliation, dignity and self-respect. *Philosophical Psychology* 13 (4): 523–40.

Street, A. F., and D. W. Kissane. 2001. Constructions of dignity in end-of-life care. *Journal of Palliative Care* 17 (2): 93–101.

Sulmasy, D. P. 2007. Human Dignity and Human Worth. In *Perspectives on Human Dignity: A Conversation*, edited by J. Malpas and N. Lickis, 9–18. Dordrecht, Netherlands: Springer.

Sulmasy, D. P. 2008. Dignity and Bioethics. In *Human Dignity and Bioethics: Essays Commissioned by the President's Council on Bioethics*, 469–501. Washington, DC: President's Council on Bioethics.

Szawarski, Z. 1986. Dignity and responsibility. *Dialectics and Humanism* 2/3: 193–205.

Tadd, W., and M. Calnan. 2009. Caring for older people: Why dignity matters—the European experience. In *Dignity in Care for Older People*, edited by L. Nordenfelt, 119–45. Chichester, UK: Wiley-Blackwell.

Tamayo-Acosta, J. J. 2003. Dignity and Liberation: A Theological and Political Perspective. In *The Discourse of Human Dignity*, edited by R. Ammicht-Quinn, M. Junker-Kenny, and E. Tamez, 67–77. London: SCM Press.

Tarantola, D. 2000. Building on the Synergy between Health and Human Rights: A Global Perspective. François-Xavier Bagnoud Center for Health and Human Rights Working Paper Series, No. 8. Boston: Harvard School of Public Health.

Tattersall, M. 2007. Dignity and Health. In *Perspectives on Human Dignity:*

A Conversation, edited by J. Malpas and N. Lickis, 187–91. Dordrecht, Netherlands: Springer.

Thomas, J. E. 2000. Incorporating empowerment into models of care: Strategies from feminist women's health centers. *Research in the Sociology of Health Care* 17: 139–52.

Tinder, G. 2003. Facets of personal dignity. In *In Defense of Human Dignity: Essays for Our Times*, edited by R. P. Kraynak and G. Tinder, 237–45. Notre Dame, IN: University of Notre Dame Press.

Truss, L. 2005. *Talk to the Hand*. New York: Gotham Books.

Tunstall, W. W. 1985. Dignity: A Psychological Construct. PhD diss., Virginia Commonwealth University.

Tuomi, M. T. 2001. *Human Dignity in the Learning Environment*. Jyväskylä, Finland: Institute for Educational Research.

United States Department of Justice, Office of Legal Counsel. 2002a. *Memorandum for Alberto R. Gonzalez, Counsel to the President, Re: Standards of Conduct for Interrogation under 18 USC 2340-2340A*. *www.aclu.org/accountability/olc.html*.

United States Department of Justice, Office of Legal Counsel. 2002b. *Memorandum for John Rizzo, Acting General Counsel of the Central Intelligence Agency: Interrogation of al Qaeda Operative*. *www.aclu.org/accountability/olc.html*.

United States Department of Justice, Office of the Inspector General. 2008. *A Review of the FBI's Involvement in and Observations of Detainee Interrogations in Guantanamo Bay, Afghanistan, and Iraq*. Washington, DC: Oversight and Review Division Office of the Inspector General.

United States Senate Committee on Armed Services. 2008. *Inquiry into the Treatment of Detainees in US Custody*. *armed-services.senate.gov*.

Universal Declaration of Human Rights. 1948. Adopted and proclaimed by United Nations General Assembly Resolution 217A (III), December 10. *www.un.org/en/documents/udhr/*.

Valadier, P. 2003. The Person Who Lacks Dignity. In *The Discourse of Human Dignity*, edited by R. Ammicht-Quinn, M. Junker-Kenny, and E. Tamez, 49–56. London: SCM Press.

Valentine, N., C. Darby, and G. J. Bonsel. 2008. Which aspects of non-clinical quality of care are most important? Results from WHO's general population surveys of "health system responsiveness" in 41 countries. *Social Science and Medicine* 66 (9): 1939–50.

Wainwright, P., and A. Gallagher. 2008. On different types of dignity in nursing care: A critique of Nordenfelt. *Nursing Philosophy* 9: 46–54.

Waskul, D. D., and P. van der Riet. 2002. The abject embodiment of cancer patients: Dignity, selfhood, and the grotesque body. *Symbolic Interaction* 25 (4): 487–513.

Wenk-Ansohn, M. 2001. The Vestige of Pain. In *At the Side of Torture Survivors*, edited by S. Graessner, N. Gurris, and C. Pross, and translated by J. M. Riemer, 57–69. Baltimore: Johns Hopkins University Press.

Werner, A., and K. Malterud. 2003. It is hard work behaving as a credible patient: Encounters between women with chronic pain and their doctors. *Social Science and Medicine* 57 (8): 1409–19.

Wilkinson, R. G. 1999. Putting the Picture Together: Prosperity, Redistribution, Health and Welfare. In *Social Determinants of Health*, edited by M. Marmot and R. G. Wilkinson, 256–74. Oxford: Oxford University Press.

Wilkinson, R. G. 2005. *The Impact of Inequality: How to Make Sick Societies Healthier.* London: Routledge.

Wilkinson, R. G., and K. Pickett. 2009. *The Spirit Level: Why Greater Equality Makes Societies Stronger.* New York: Bloomsbury Press.

Wilkinson, R. G., and K. Pickett. 2010. *Reply to Critics.* London: Equality Trust. equalitytrust.org.uk.

Witte, J., Jr. 2003. Between Sanctity and Depravity: Human Dignity in Protestant Perspective. In *In Defense of Human Dignity: Essays for Our Times*, edited by R. P. Kraynak and G. Tinder, 119–37. Notre Dame, IN: University of Notre Dame Press.

Woogara, J. 2005. Patients' privacy of the person and human rights. *Nursing Ethics* 12 (3): 273–87.

Woolhead, G., W. Tadd, J. A. Boix-Ferrer, S. Krajcik, B. Schmid-Pfahler, B. Spjuth, D. Stratton, and P. Dieppe. 2006. "Tu" or "Vous"? A European qualitative study of dignity and communication with older people in health and social care settings. *Patient Education and Counseling* 61 (3): 363–71.

World Health Organization. 1948. Preamble to the Constitution of the World Health Organization as adopted by the International Health Conference, New York, June 19–July 22, 1946; signed on July 22, 1946 by the representatives of 61 States (Official Records of the World Health Organization, no. 2, p. 100) and entered into force on April 7, 1948. *www.who.int.*

Yamin, A. A. 2009. Shades of dignity: Exploring the demands of equality in applying human rights frameworks to health. *Health and Human Rights* 11 (2): 1–18.

Zhang, Q. 2000. The idea of human dignity in classical Chinese philosophy: A reconstruction of Confucianism. *Journal of Chinese Philosophy* 27 (3): 299–330.

INDEX